Women in Veterinary Medicine

Women
IN VETERINARY MEDICINE
Profiles of Success

Dr. Sue Drum

Dr. H. Ellen Whiteley

Iowa State University Press / Ames

Dr. Sue Drum, who practiced small-animal medicine for twenty-five years, is the state veterinarian for Fox Valley Greyhound Track, Kaukauna, Wisconsin.

Dr. H. Ellen Whiteley owns and operates a house-call service for cats in Amarillo, Texas. She also owns a public relations business.

Authorization to photocopy items for internal or personal use, or the internal or personal use of specific clients, is granted by Iowa State University Press, provided that the base fee of $.10 per copy is paid directly to the Copyright Clearance Center, 27 Congress Street, Salem, MA 01970. For those organizations that have been granted a photocopy license by CCC, a separate system of payments has been arranged. The fee codes for users of the Transactional Reporting Service are 0-8138-0668-2/91 $.10.

⊗ Printed on acid-free paper in the United States of America

First edition, 1991

Library of Congress Cataloging-in-Publication Data

Drum, Sue
    Women in veterinary medicine: profiles of success / Sue Drum, H. Ellen Whiteley.—1st ed.
        p.   cm.
    ISBN 0-8138-0668-2 (alk. paper)
    1. Women veterinarians—United States—Biography. 2. Veterinarians—United States—Biography. I. Whiteley, H. Ellen. II. Title.
    [DNLM: 1. Veterinary Medicine—biography. 2. Women—biography. WZ 112 D795w]
    SF612.D78 1991
    636.089'092'2—dc20
    [B]
    DNLM/DLC
    for Library of Congress   91-7050

WE DEDICATE THIS BOOK

to the twenty professional women

who graciously shared their

lives and thoughts with us

and who provide exciting lessons

in courage and self-determination.

CONTENTS

PREFACE

by H. Ellen Whiteley

T he idea for a book about female veterinarians was born separately in each of us coauthors. It is perhaps a miracle that we found each other—we live in different areas of the country and have never met, except through correspondence and telephone conversations. Yet we managed, in spite of those geographical handicaps and different writing styles, to coauthor this book.

You may detect diverging voices and approaches as you read these twenty profiles. We hope that you overlook our disparities and enjoy and learn from each woman's experiences in a profession once considered a male domain.

As we began to select women for this book, it quickly became apparent that we could not interview every woman who has made significant contributions to veterinary medicine, nor could we adequately chronicle the contributions that women now deceased have made to our profession. We were also aware that thousands of female veterinarians, receiving few awards or accolades, were quietly working at their chosen occupation, doing a good job, and contributing to society. We are all shaping the profession.

The women who were interviewed spanned three generations. In spite of our age differences, we share many parallels. Fifteen of us are firstborn or only children. Firstborns and only children have been described as perfectionistic, reliable, conscientious, loyal, goal-oriented, achievement-oriented, people-pleasing, self-sacrificing, and self-reliant. Dr. Kevin Leman, the author of *The Birth Order Book,* writes, "Firstborns typically go for anything that takes precision, strong powers of concentration, and dogged mental discipline. A much greater proportion of firstborns wind up in 'high achievement' professions such as science, medicine, or law." Dr. Leman describes only children as super-firstborns.

We can take that characteristic of dogged mental discipline and extrapolate it to mean dogged determination. The women in this book do not take no for an answer. In fact, the challenge of "You can't do that" was irresistible to many of us. Several women stated that gender discrimination made them stronger and more focused toward their goals.

But who are we as people? We are just like other women. We are daughters, wives, and mothers. We are also single, divorced, and widowed. We are more apt to suffer from the superwoman syndrome than from the Cinderella complex. In other words, we tend to care for others and to take charge of our destiny rather than wait for external forces to transform our lives.

We come from rural, urban, and suburban settings. Our parents are professionals, white-collar workers, and blue-collar workers. Most of us had strong father role models who often served as our first mentors. For some of us, home elicits memories of family dinners and a nurturing family, but others of us are the adult survivors of families suffering from mental illness, alcoholism, and incest. We were shaped by our early experiences but not defined by them.

We have strong and often dissimilar values. We may be animal rightists or animal researchers, vegetarians or meat eaters, members of traditional religions or adherents of New Age spirituality. We share concerns about overpopulation and the environment. Money is not our primary motivator. We are driven by an internal value system. We want to make a difference.

And we do make a difference. Since 1983, female applicants to U.S. schools of veterinary medicine have outnumbered male applicants. It is projected that by the turn of the century approximately 33 percent of the veterinarians in this country will be female. In spite of problems forecast for the profession, such as low salaries, government restrictions, and reduced livestock operations, we will find creative solutions and we will persevere. It's our nature.

INTRODUCTION

by Sue Drum

W hen the first veterinary schools were created in 1762, it was thought that all veterinarians would be men. This view was understandable, because most graduates earned their living during long hours in dark, drafty barns or stables, treating sick horses and cows that required great strength to restrain and medicate. As late as the 1970s, educated men and women believed that a woman could not practice veterinary medicine and remain "a lady." In fact, many believed that women did not belong in any profession, let alone one as rugged as veterinary medicine.

In the early days, a few very determined women did graduate from veterinary school. Aleen Cust, the first female graduate, completed her training at the Royal Veterinary College in Edinburgh, Scotland, in 1900. However, because of her sex, she was not allowed to write the final exam and was denied her degree. For more than twenty years Cust worked actively in her profession, and in 1922, at age fifty-four, she was finally allowed to take the exam and receive her degree. Little is known about the first female veterinarian in the United States, Mignon Nicholson, who graduated from McKillip College in 1903. In 1910 two more women received doctor of veterinary medicine (D.V.M.) degrees, Elinor McGrath from Chicago College and Florence Kimball from Cornell University. McGrath practiced small-animal medicine successfully until she retired in 1947.

By 1936 there were 30 female veterinarians in the United States. These women had to be superachievers, because admission to veterinary college for a woman was nearly impossible. By earning undergraduate and often graduate degrees before entering veterinary schools, women had to prove beyond doubt their fortitude for a veterinary career. In contrast, men in the early twentieth century were accepted directly from high school, and it wasn't until 1949 that two years of preveterinary training was required for entrance to the four-year veterinary colleges. By 1970 most veterinary colleges required three and usually four years of preveterinary credits.

In 1963 there were 277 female veterinarians in the United States, a mere fraction of the total profession. As long as female numbers remained small, the profession felt no threat and saw no need to ponder problems women might cause. But when 15 qualified women appeared in the 1962 freshman class at the University of Illinois, mild shock waves had stirred the faculty. Should there be a limit to the number of women accepted? What would taxpayers say when these women stayed home to raise a family and never used their education? The veterinary curriculum was designed to serve agriculture. Would women be acceptable on the farm? Wasn't strength the real issue? Large-animal medicine was just too physical for a woman, the faculty thought.

In 1963 the American Veterinary Medical Association published a study that predicted a need for twice the number of veterinarians in the next twenty years. As veterinary schools expanded, so did the number of female veterinarians. Seven new veterinary colleges opened their doors between 1970 and 1985. As the popularity of the profession peaked, 8 students applied for every opening. In just ten years, from 1976 to 1986, total student enrollment increased by 2,648. During the same ten years, the number of female students increased by 3,397, until women made up 51.5 percent of the graduating classes. Women not only filled all new openings but also were supplanting men in significant numbers.

In 1987 women made up 17 percent of the veterinary profession as a whole, and 22 percent in 1989, but their numbers in veterinary school rose to 60 percent. Never had such a male-dominated profession experienced such a great influx of women in so short a time. As American workplaces become feminized at a much slower rate, the veterinary profession becomes a cultural prophet, offering a unique insight into a world where women gain authority.

Why did veterinary colleges suddenly open their doors to women? Federal legislation and the women's movement paved the way. The Equal Pay Act of 1963 and the Civil Rights Act of 1964 guaranteed equal opportunity in training, hiring, promotion, and pay regardless of sex, race, color, religion, or national origin.

The education amendments of 1972 and the Women's Educational Act of 1974 prevented sex discrimination by educational institutions receiving federal funds. Veterinary colleges had managed to gain access to sizable sums of federal money and influence only recently, in 1966, so they bent over backwards not to discriminate. With the barriers removed, the number of women entering veterinary school doubled in 1975, and women continue to flood the profession.

The increase of women in the general work force was influenced by the women's movement, which made a career acceptable, and by the economy, which made two incomes necessary for families trying to maintain their middle-class standard of living. Still, why did so many women want to be veterinarians? Although no one claims to have the exact answer, possibilities abound.

New anesthetics and tranquilizers make brawn less essential on the farm than it used to be. Even male veterinarians find that their productive years are drastically shortened by wrestling steers, roping horses, and chasing pigs. Imbued with new self-esteem, livestock veterinarians are abandoning the image of the raw cowboy for that of a competent, qualified diagnostician. Small-animal medicine continues to expand as numerous modern pet clinics are built. Certainly a woman can handle a ten-pound cat as well as a man can.

By tradition a woman is often labeled as being more sensitive than a man. Yet it was a man, James Herriot, who portrayed the relationship between patient and veterinarian with warmth and humor. Many people believe that his books, published in the early 1970s, added greatly to the profession's popularity.

Lulled by a romantic view of herself easing the suffering of animals, a young woman was often blind to the problems of excelling. After eight years in college to master a plethora of rigorous courses relevant to seven animal species, the new graduate had to decide if she wanted to pursue her career while she raised a family. In her mid-twenties when she graduated, she knew that children would take time away from her career.

Although the majority of veterinary women today choose to combine career and marriage, almost half (49 percent) choose not to have children. Those women who do have children usually have only one or two and are older than the general population—around thirty—when their first child is born.

According to research by Patricia Cawunder at Northwestern University, veterinary students in 1971 believed more strongly in the stereotypic male and female roles than law students did. The moderately masculine self-concept enjoyed by law students of both sexes was a great advantage to the female because she did not worry about fulfilling the traditional family role. In contrast, the married veterinary woman tried to be a perfect homemaker and mother even if her husband was understanding and supportive of her career.

The differences between female lawyers and female veterinarians could in part be due to the difference between growing up in a city and growing up in the country. Most veterinarians come from small towns where traditional values are well ingrained. Whatever the answer, trying to juggle both career and family causes stress on both partners, and the divorce rate among veterinarians is considerably higher than the national average.

Although women continue to flock to veterinary school, young men are turning to careers that offer greater earning potential. Starting salaries for veterinarians have not kept pace with the cost of living. In 1980 the average starting salary was $17,175, and in 1988 it was $22,181. In real terms, when these salaries are corrected for the cost of living, graduates' average starting salaries declined from $20,768 in 1980 to $18,699 in 1988, a 10 percent decrease in purchasing power. The starting salaries for physicians are almost three times higher, and veterinarians who believe that their expertise is equal to that of physicians chafe at the knowledge that they can charge only one-tenth of their counterparts' fees. Engineering, computer science, and a host of other careers that require less time and money to learn also offer greater financial security.

Women don't seem to be as concerned about low pay as men are, and it is that viewpoint that worries men most. Will feminization keep veterinary income low? The average starting salaries for women are $1,000 less than those for men. One reason is the large number of women in small-animal practice and university teaching, the two areas with the lowest incomes. But the problem of long hours for low pay has plagued the profession from its inception. Women did not cause this image problem. A 1934 article in *Veterinary Medicine* by editor D. M. Campbell noted, "Despite its important achievements and obvious merit, little is known about veterinary medicine and even less appreciated by the general public and by agriculture which it serves."

New to the idea of being self-supporting and being the

family breadwinner, the female veterinarian has to overcome old feelings of inferiority. To undervalue her own worth, to regard her profession as a hobby or a second income, to follow her husband's career rather than her own, will indeed lower her salary and image. Today's average female veterinarian projects a healthy self-image, however. She is thirty-four, is married, has completed eight years of college, holds an undergraduate degree as well as her D.V.M., works full-time in her profession with only a short leave of absence to have a baby, and feels compelled to take care of her home and children as well as her career. Her average income is $29,600 per year, whereas that of the average male veterinarian is $50,300 per year.

Female veterinarians as a whole are younger than their male counterparts, but they are coming of age and standing on the threshold of positions of influence. Several now appear among the policymakers in the American Veterinary Medical Association and the American Animal Hospital Association. The Women's Veterinary Medical Association provides intelligent support, patiently urging "Give the woman a chance," and more men are following that advice. Women are publishing in scientific journals, are serving on faculties of veterinary colleges, and are prominent in practice specialty groups. As women seek greater responsibility, men become more accustomed to their presence.

In the next twenty years women will gain more authority in the veterinary hierarchy. Will they find solutions that men failed to consider? Can there ever be too many educated minds, too many good ideas, too much honest concern? If future generations of female veterinarians spring from the same fertile seed as the women in this book, men's fears about them will prove false.

Most of the information in the introduction is based on a 1987 honors thesis, "Women in the Veterinary Profession: Yesterday and Today," by Lauralyn J. Brown, a fourth-year preveterinary student at Hampshire College, Amherst, Massachusetts. The thesis includes a lengthy and complete bibliography.

I am especially indebted to Mary Ellen Pourchot, my wonderful writing teacher and critic who, in the course of this book, became my friend.
Sue Drum

Women in Veterinary Medicine

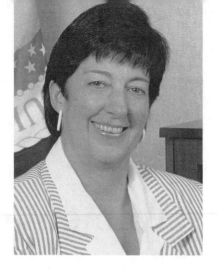

Joan Arnoldi

JOAN ARNOLDI'S early career established her as one of the most prominent small-animal practitioners in Wisconsin. She seemed to be directing every major issue in the state's veterinary profession. Before long, she was the first female state veterinarian in Wisconsin and, for that matter, in the United States.

A graduate of the University of Illinois College of Veterinary Medicine, Arnoldi received her doctor of veterinary medicine degree in 1963. Previously she had earned a bachelor of science in zoology (1956) and a master of science in physiology (1959).

In the 1960s Arnoldi established the first successful pet practice in rural Wausau, Wisconsin. By the 1970s, practitioners were referring difficult small-animal surgeries to Arnoldi and seeking her expertise in feline medicine. Arnoldi was active in the American Association of Feline Practitioners from 1974 and sat on its executive board from 1979 to 1986, serving as president for two years. Today she is on the advisory council to Cornell Feline Health Center and is a member of the American Veterinary Medical Association's house of delegates for the American Association

of Feline Practitioners.

In 1971 Arnoldi became the first woman on the Wisconsin State Board of Veterinary Examiners and served an unprecedented three terms (1971 to 1984), having been appointed by three separate governors. In 1977 Arnoldi, elected to a three-year term, was the only woman on the National Board of Veterinary Examiners. From 1977 to 1981 Arnoldi was on the executive board of the American Association of Veterinary State Boards, serving as president of the association one year.

Supporting a program to train animal technicians from its inception in the early 1970s, Arnoldi wrote the original legislation in the Wisconsin Veterinary Practice Act that regulated the use of animal technicians. The act allowed Wisconsin animal technicians to practice under veterinary supervision with more freedom than technicians enjoyed in any other state.

Arnoldi joined the planning committee for a veterinary college on the Madison campus of the University of Wisconsin in the late 1970s. She was determined to help build and staff the best possible facility.

In 1980 Arnoldi became the director

of the Bureau of Technical Services in the Animal Health Division of Wisconsin's Department of Agriculture, Trade, and Consumer Protection, with responsibility for the Central Animal Health Laboratory and regional laboratories.

Arnoldi became chief administrator of the Animal Health Division in the Wisconsin Department of Agriculture in 1984. In that position she made history as the first female state veterinarian in the nation.

In 1989 Arnoldi became the first female veterinarian in the senior executive service of the U.S. Department of Agriculture, Division of Animal and Plant Health Inspection Service, as deputy administrator for a new agency called Regulatory Enforcement and Animal Care. Arnoldi was also the first woman to be elected, in 1986, as an officer of the prestigious United States Animal Health Association; she had served since 1984 as the only woman on its executive committee. Also in 1986, Arnoldi was elected president of the Wisconsin Council of the Professions. "I'm the kind of person who accepts the risk of a new challenge," she says. "Of course, someday I may become involved in something I can't handle, but that's the thrill of the risk."

Recently Arnoldi attended the Tenth Annual Symposium on Veterinary Medical Education in Michigan to head a workshop on the demographics of women in veterinary medicine. She expected to confront the usual group of senior men, probably deans of veterinary colleges. "What a pleasant surprise," she says, "to find my workshop populated with bright young women, not one man. These women, who had graduated from classrooms filled with a comfortable number of women, were imbued with the excitement of practice and academics. They did not sense the struggle ahead for their gender to gain positions of leadership. As more women enter the veterinary profession, they must take an interest in their professional organizations. They must be willing to assume a dominant role or, as male veterinarians decrease in number, our profession will have a leadership void. If only men seek authority, some of the best minds will not be in the right places."

Attracted to positions of power and responsibility, Joan Arnoldi continues to lay fresh tracks for women to follow.

■

I've always believed strongly in myself. I had to. I was the first person in my family to go to college. My relatives could not understand why I needed so much education. Work was more honorable, they thought. Until I left the University of Illinois after ten years and became employed, I was the family black sheep.

In my early school days I was a good student with a science interest, and several teachers encouraged me to go to college. The most educated and respected person I knew was our family doctor, so I patterned myself after him. I enrolled at the University of Illinois in premedicine. My father encouraged me to be a doctor, but my mother thought I should choose a feminine career like nursing or teaching.

That first year, the battle to get into medical school overwhelmed me. The men, who studied together and helped each other in their medical fraternity, were not friendly to female competition. In my second year I changed to zoology.

I grew up with a sincere love of animals. In family photographs, from toddler on, I'm the skinny girl, holding the cat. My family lived in Belvidere, Illinois, which was then quite countrylike, and I was encouraged to keep pets. Like other children, I had chickens and rabbits and cats and dogs. I was so fascinated by my pets that instead of joining school groups, I spent a great deal of time with animals. My sister, who was seven years older and into ballet, called me a tomboy.

When I graduated with my bachelor of science in zoology, I accepted a job with G. D. Searle in medical research. I worked in its cardiac unit, testing new heart drugs on dogs. Research was very satisfying, but I immediately saw that I needed a master's degree to advance. After one year, I was back at the University of Illinois, studying mammalian physiology with a job waiting for me at Searle's when I'd earned my degree.

Norbert Arnoldi was my classmate, and we began dating. By the second year, all my plans had changed. Norbert and I would marry after graduation and enter the College of Veterinary Medicine at Illinois to prepare for a career we both wanted. This was the first time I pictured myself seriously as a veterinarian.

Freshman year in the veterinary college, Norbert and I had a light course load, since we'd already completed difficult subjects like biochemistry. We were both able to work part-time for the university, and our finances, always low, began to grow. Soon I realized I was pregnant, but even dissecting preserved animals in anatomy class was no bother. Pleased with our career choice and in control of our time, we looked forward to becoming parents.

Our son was born with severe congenital defects, the worst being hydrocephalus. Those first hours after delivery drained our emotions. Later I felt strongly that it was my duty to stay home and care for my son. Norb and my father insisted I stay in class. They understood, better than I, that my education would hold me together. When the dean of the veterinary school became aware of our struggle, he graciously placed our son at the University of Illinois Research Hospital. There our child received the best possible care until, at age four, he died.

My father's death, near the end of my second year, only added to the unpleasant memory of my student days. My grades were low, but with the soothing assurance of friends and my strong husband to lean on, I found the strength to pass. There were other students who didn't. Starting with a class of forty-one, only twenty-seven, including all three women, received their doctor of veterinary medicine degree.

After graduation, Norbert and I joined a group practice in Edwardsville, Illinois. One year later, with a little money in our pockets, we dared to stop work and tour Wisconsin, camping out most nights, while we searched for a good place for Norbert to build a dairy practice. Soon we heard about a veterinarian in Wausau who wanted to leave after fifteen years in practice and work for the state. He offered us an affordable deal—pay for the drugs and equipment and rent his clinic, a big red barn. We accepted, and his farm clients immediately switched their affection to Norb and kept him busy day and night treating cattle.

In charge of organizing the barn, I decided to build a small-animal practice. My first day at work, I scheduled a spay but couldn't find a scalpel. As the ex-proprietor departed, he suggested I hold a blade in my hand as he had done. Then I knew clearly I would be starting from scratch. Neighboring livestock veterinarians warned me that in farm country, people didn't invest in medical care for dogs and cats. One year later I had redecorated and reorganized the barn until it resembled a suitable pet clinic. Then I called Wausau Homes and asked for help in designing a new, prefabricated veterinary hospital.

After two and a half years in the barn, we moved to our new building, designed and equipped according to modern guidelines from the American Animal Hospital Association. We had ample space for small-animal patients and even room for Norbert's farm patients and supplies. The move prompted a growth spurt in my practice, and I trained four young women as animal technicians to help me. After three years the demand for pet care was more than I could handle. Norb and I hired a veterinary associate to take over the country work so Norb could help me in the hospital. More sociable than I, Norb examined dogs and cats and chatted with the clients while I concentrated on surgery. My colleagues would say to me, "Don't you get sick of spaying dogs? It's the same routine, over and over." I never felt that way. To me there were enough variables, old dogs, fat dogs, dogs with weak hearts, to make each spay a little different.

As our practice grew, I continued to handle all administrative duties, hiring, firing, teaching and motivating our staff, and controlling finances. Eventually we had thirteen employees, four of them veterinarians.

Norbert and I were so enthusiastic about veterinary medicine that it consumed our free time together. We shared animal stories and discussed business. At a local professional meeting a veterinarian cornered me to tell me how his long hours at work drove his wife crazy.

"Now, you"—he pointed knowingly—"being a veterinarian, must be sympathetic to your husband!"

"No," I told him, "I get mad too when he's late for dinner." It was strange, but Norb's long hours irritated me more than my own.

When we first started practice and lay exhausted from the daily struggle, we talked about looking for separate jobs in Chicago and making more money with less effort. Then we'd agree that the struggle was teaching us things we could never learn working for someone else.

One of us was always on emergency call, so we had no social life. Instead we bought forty acres outside Wausau and raised sheep, butchering the lambs for our own meat. This hobby ended when our sheep escaped and spread out over the country one too many times. We never found a fence that could contain sheep.

One of my clients gave me an Abyssinian kitten, and in no time I was hooked on that breed. I built a colony of twenty-five cats and traveled around the country entering my cats in shows. It was a nice escape from practice. By talking to cat breeders, I learned a great deal about cattery medicine, which is entirely different from treating the individual pet. Cattery problems did not interest most veterinarians, so before long I was sought as a feline specialist. I joined the American Association of Feline Practitioners and served on its executive board for seven years. As my career has changed, I've kept up on feline medicine. I've even found a little time for research on feline diseases and have published my findings in several scientific papers. I still have as pets four aging remnants from my cat colony.

As our practice continued to profit, Norbert and I at last had time to ourselves. We bought a twenty-four-foot cabin cruiser that slept six, and we learned to sail. By then we could take vacations together. With friends we sailed Lake Superior and Lake Winnebago. We bought a home on a four-acre, wooded peninsula in

Lake Wausau. It was only five miles from the practice, but surrounded by other islands, it felt like the middle of nowhere.

After nineteen years of marriage, Norbert and I were divorced. It was time for me to leave the practice. As much as I enjoyed my clients, I never intended to practice all my life. I still feel that if a person is going to make a contribution to a chosen career area, it will probably be within five to seven years. I was anxious for change.

Until then, my profession had accepted me as Norbert's wife. Now people would have to take me at face value. Free of family obligations, my choice of jobs was unlimited. I could possibly study small-animal surgery for five years and become a board-certified surgeon, or seek work in private industry or even in government. Until I decided, I accepted a part-time position in Madison at the state diagnostic laboratory. I handled abortions in dairy cattle and necropsied fetuses to become reacquainted with large-animal medicine.

When the year was over, I accepted an offer from Pitman-Moore in New Jersey to become senior research clinician. My work for this private drug company required travel to veterinary schools and to some private practices to set up clinical testing trials for new drugs. A year later Wisconsin's Department of Agriculture asked me to interview for the job of director of the Bureau of Technical Services. When I was chosen, I became one of the first women in this high management position. The agriculture and livestock industry was always considered male territory. I would administer not only the Central Animal Health Laboratory, where I had worked, but also the regional laboratories. My twelve years on the State Board of Veterinary Examiners had prepared me for this position. As a board member, I helped prepare and administer the state licensing exam, with questions on all animal species but with emphasis on livestock. This duty kept me current and in touch with the needs of agriculture.

As an administrator, I had several management courses to my credit, but my most useful skills were those I'd developed operating my small-animal practice. In state government I learned a great deal on the job from my staff veterinarians with advanced degrees in pathology, virology, and parasitology and from my boss, Dr. Willis Lyle. Dr. Lyle was my teacher and my friend. When he died, I lost an irreplaceable ally.

To fill Dr. Lyle's position as chief administrator of the Animal Health Division, I was one of several candidates interviewed by the secretary of agriculture. In February 1984, I was appointed the first woman state veterinarian, not only in Wisconsin but in the United States. I had overcome the common viewpoint that women would ruin the profession because they "lacked upper-body strength." Veterinarians were still concerned that women, as a group, would have no interest in agriculture, but as I assumed the highest agricultural state office a veterinarian could occupy, I was warmly welcomed.

A subtle change accompanied my elevated status. I lost civil service protection. Instead I served at the pleasure of the secretary of agriculture. He could fire me whenever he wished. I tried hard to please my boss.

Like an ant in a sugar factory, I found many tempting opportunities. The era of tough, do-as-we-say-or-else state law enforcement was closing as cigar-puffing, old-time livestock veterinarians reached retirement age. Their tough strategy had rid Wisconsin of diseases like tuberculosis and brucellosis and left a sound system of surveillance in place.

To initiate a new government attitude of cooperation and compromise with the livestock producer, I hired agreeable veterinarians still in their prime. I'd left behind a good team at the diagnostic laboratory, and with my present staff in place I immediately focused everyone's attention on building a usable pilot program for eradication of pseudorabies. Wisconsin, I realized, presented an ideal testing ground because we had outlawed the use of pseudorabies vaccine. Without vaccinated pigs to confuse the results of blood testing, carrier pigs could be clearly identified. Wisconsin became one of five states funded by the federal government to effect a model program.

My staff and I tried first to win the cooperation of swine producers by convincing them that eradication of pseudorabies would eventually mean more money in their pocket. Pseudorabies is a disease caused by a herpesvirus. There is no effective treatment. Baby pigs rarely survive, but older pigs can resist or overcome the disease and become carriers. Even pigs that appear healthy can shed the virus and act as a source of infection for other pigs, cattle, and even dogs and cats. When animals other than pigs are infected, these animals die within a few days. If we could eradicate the virus from swine herds, not only pigs would be protected but other livestock and pets as well.

My field veterinarians hoped to test blood from every pig in Wisconsin. I attended local farm meetings with my veterinarians and explained our test-and-eliminate program. At one meeting a reporter baited me sarcastically, "Do you think these farmers are going to allow the state to march onto their private property?" In the old days farmers were known to chase state agents off their land with shotguns. Now we needed the farmers' cooperation. We encouraged swine producers to air their gripes and help us construct a workable program.

Swine blood tubes began to appear at our diagnostic laboratory and eventually eighteen herds in Wisconsin were quarantined. Pseudorabies was present in these herds, and the farmer was given two years to remove all infected pigs. Our rules were lenient. We even allowed producers to market infected herds to cut their loss. After two years, Wisconsin had only eleven quarantined herds. We don't know how long it will take for total eradication, but until this is accomplished I will work hard to keep this program on track. I must keep my staff motivated, find intelligent answers to producers' complaints, and most important, continue to believe that this program will work.

Meanwhile I have to deal with other problems. The farm crisis is real, and it's not over yet. When a small town's economy is hurt and its banks fail, this disaster eventually mushrooms to affect metropolitan areas. The state provides counseling not only for bankrupt farmers but also for companies dealing with these farmers, like utilities and banks.

I'm also concerned with the foreign export market for livestock and animal products. Agribusiness relies on foreign sales, and I must keep track of the ever-changing import requirements. Live cattle or any products from cattle that test positive for the disease bovine leukosis cannot be exported. To increase exports, I've begun a voluntary blood testing program that certifies cattle free of bovine leukosis.

Being a horse person with my own forty-acre Arabian horse farm, I enjoy helping other horse breeders. All horses imported from foreign countries are held in quarantine until repeated tests prove they are free of the disease equine infectious metritis. The nearest quarantine station in the past was in Kentucky, where Wisconsin horses languished for six months, too far away for their owners to supervise or train. My department established three quarantine stations in Wisconsin and made our horse breeders happy.

The new veterinary college at Madison accepted its first student class in 1983. Taking office just a year later, I was able to coordinate our animal health services with theirs to avoid duplication and save money. I was given the title of adjunct assistant professor. Later I was promoted to adjunct associate professor. Actually I was an adviser in pathobiology, and veterinary student rotation was scheduled through the state health laboratory. Twice a year I lectured to veterinary students, hoping to inspire a few to choose regulatory medicine. After one lecture two young men told me that out of the entire student body—over three hundred—they were the only two interested in regulatory medicine. Students haven't changed much. When I was in school, any classmate considering regulatory medicine was considered weird.

Students are interested in humane treatment of animals. At one time I was state humane officer and could feel the hot breath of animal rights activists on my neck. These groups are well funded and getting stronger. They push legislation based on considerable misinformation. If veterinarians and livestock producers don't use their knowledge to solve some of the abuse problems, foolish laws harmful to agriculture will be passed.

Presently, my time is consumed by revising the unintelligible book of regulations I administer. Since 1930, state laws governing animal health have been added a piece at a time, and it's almost impossible to find one clear thought. When a farmer asks me to interpret some outdated regulation, I'm embarrassed. So I'm rewriting the regulations into reasonable, everyday language. Some farmers and veterinarians don't understand why a foolish rule takes so long to correct. They aren't aware of Wisconsin's unique open form of government, which makes state residents the decision makers. Every regulation I rewrite passes through government committees to the legislature for revision. Then it's presented at five or six public hearings to add opinions from the general public and all their special-interest groups. What comes back to me is an alien rule. I rewrite, cognizant of public opinion, and relaunch. Eventually a revised law is passed. This is easily a five-year project. The public forum system is burdensome, but in a way you have to admire it. I certainly can't contrive something behind closed doors and lay it on an unsuspecting public. When regulations are passed, they are acceptable to the majority of those affected.

In private practice I could make quick, easy decisions. In government I adhere to rigid policy. Direct action is rare. But I have learned to accept the paper flow, the endless meetings, the waste of time. My every move and decision are based on sound scientific evidence. I am no longer frustrated when people don't see things my way. I've grown patient. I tell myself, "Hey! I believe in what I'm doing. I can hang on to this idea a long time if I have to."

I never want to become a pure bureaucrat, a person who caves into the system and stops making waves. If an employee has no experience in free enterprise, he won't fight bureaucracy. Parts of the system I must accept, like budget, protocol, political pressure, but I don't have to accept everything. There are many little imperfections I try to change. These small accomplishments accumulate. Once in a while I can even take direct action. A big-name dairy producer calls the local assemblyperson and complains because Wisconsin is the only state in the country that won't allow semen from the nation's top jersey bull to be used. The bull tests positive for Johne's disease, a disease we are attempting to control, but the infecting organism is not in the semen. The semen is harmless. The assemblyperson calls me directly, and I waive the rule. Behind the scenes, I spend hours checking the testing protocol on that semen to be sure it really is safe. Quick decisions are fun unless they're wrong.

People always want government to do more for less money. This is a challenge to my animal health department. I am responsible for the animal health budget. We do more belt tightening than wasteful spending.

I don't plan to retire in this position. Presently I'm too involved to consider my next challenge. Certainly I hold no illusion of returning to practice, even though I miss the close personal contact. There is so much new information in every aspect of medicine. It's too much to relearn. I am no longer involved with individual animals but rather entire herds and populations. As I move further into government, I grow more narrow and have fewer choices. When I graduated, I was a generalist. I was informed on all the animal species. I could choose practice or research. I chose small-animal practice, then small-animal surgery, then diagnostic medicine, regulatory medicine, and finally pure administration. I may be the first woman through many doors, but I don't consider myself interesting. I would not sparkle at a cocktail party. Veterinarians and students are intrigued by my varied career, but outside my profession I'm only good for small talk on pets.

I attract attention because women aren't supposed to be interested in agriculture. Actually there is no job unsuited to a woman. I used to think there were limits, but women have proved me wrong. In government we are told that if all qualifications are equal, we should hire minorities. I would like to see women get more opportunity to advance. However, I hire from an approved list of applicants. The new secretary of agriculture has appointed more women than usual to this department. Still we have trouble retaining these women. Women are not given equal treatment. Obvious measurements like pay are equal. The difference is more subtle—a feeling of unevenness regarding promotion and opportunity for recognition. Women in high positions are not good to each other. They have the philosophy, "I'm climbing, you're climbing. I'm for me, you're for you." They are too insecure to help each other.

My clerical staff work well together, but they do traditional female work. Men understand the mentor system in upper management, but I have no mentor. There are no women up here. In my experience, men don't make good mentors for women. It is easier for a woman to be a mentor for a man.

I am the token woman in several prestigious organizations. The U.S. Animal Health Association, which represents veterinarians from federal, state, and industry, elected me third vice president in 1986. In five years I should move up to the rank of president. If being a woman gets my foot in the door, that's a step forward. I have to get there before I can make a difference. I don't like it when men condescend to me, but anger destroys communication. Angry women aren't welcome. I take my place among men quietly. Once my colleagues accept me, I can begin to press my ideas.

When young people ask me if they should go into veterinary medicine, I tell them the profession is very competitive and they will have to be very good at what they do. Presently veterinary schools educate students to practice. Each state requires the student to pass its board exam to become licensed. A veterinarian cannot practice or be employed in any other area of the profession—research, public health, government—without a license. In the future I see a need for more veterinarians with advanced degrees in epidemiology, pathology, and public health. This means some thoughtful restructuring of veterinary education.

Visible and vulnerable in a man's world, I draw strength from adversity. My father imprinted this trait on me when I was a child. He believed that showing emotion was a sign of weakness. I've practiced emotional control so many years that it's now a part of me. Fortunately it keeps me from bursting into tears when swine producers berate me. It also makes it very difficult to share my feelings with my friends. Sometimes I am too controlled.

In agriculture, where men are men and women are still a riddle, I have no trouble being accepted. I thought I might, and those who hired me thought I might. I am credible with livestock producers. Still, I cannot escape the female trap; if I falter, I falter not for myself but for all women. As a woman, I am on both sides of the door. I'm invited in for the feminine viewpoint and asked to leave for the same reason.

Well, it's been a year since I last talked to you, and I've been freed from my position with Wisconsin's Department of Agriculture. Now I live in Hyattsville, Maryland, and I am deputy administrator of a new agency, Regulatory Enforcement and Animal Care, which is under the Division of Animal and Plant Health Inspection Service in the U.S. Department of Agriculture.

Public sentiment, stirred by animal rights and welfare groups, has demanded stronger enforcement of the Animal Welfare Act of 1966 and its revised version in 1985. I've been building a strong enforcement arm that protects laboratory animals in biomedical research, all exhibited animals—zoo animals, roadside parks, marine mammals—and all research animals supplied by people such as dog dealers and rabbit breeders. We have a staff of veterinarians and animal technicians spread all over the country to inspect these facilities.

Our Horse Protection Act controls "sored" horses, horses on which physical or chemical devices have been used to alter the horse's natural gait. The Tennessee walking horse is the breed most involved. Ten or fifteen years ago, show spectators would see blood running down the legs of some horses. Chains were placed around the ankles, chemicals rubbed on the pasterns, and thick pads fastened under the shoes of the front feet to create the exaggerated, high-stepping gait of the walker. We've corrected this situation to a great extent, and walking-horse fans are assured that the animals have not been mistreated to achieve their exaggerated gait.

As far as animals for research are concerned, there are two views, with enormous distance in between. The research side worries that more regulation and monitoring will increase costs until research is severely limited. The far-out side doesn't want animals used for anything—research, food, clothes. Our agency tries to please the majority of people in the middle. We agree that animals should be used in research, but we want certain minimal standards enforced to improve animal treatment. With increased pressure, people in biomedical research have become very careful, basically doing their own strict monitoring.

There has been such tremendous improvement in laboratory animal care that my agency can now worry about other problems. We emphasize finding alternatives for the use of live animals and looking at new experiments very carefully to be sure they aren't duplications.

Of course, there will always be a group pushing for reform that we can't please. It is sad, but sometimes this group breaks into laboratories, smashes expensive equipment, and destroys valuable data that will take years to duplicate.

Occasionally I am harassed by individuals who want me to remedy a situation, like veal-calf husbandry, over which I have no jurisdiction. Even when I tell them I'm powerless, they aren't satisfied.

Every moment of my time is scheduled for the next six months. I like putting together a whole new structure and organization. I've always worked well with humane groups. There are people who are better administrators than I, but I am still sensitive to animal issues. With my rushed schedule, it's easy to lose this sensitivity. I must constantly remind myself what it is I'm really trying to accomplish with all my regulations. Periodically I visit my staff and observe our animal inspection procedures.

This is spring foaling season on my horse farm outside Madison. There I breed a line of pure Spanish Arabian horses, direct descendants from the strong gene pools of the Spanish military. I've spent a great deal of time securing the best stock and building a quality horse business. I still try to return to Madison for a weekend every three weeks. Then I talk to my horses and clean their stalls. It's wonderful therapy.

Someday, when this race is over, I can imagine myself with time to relax and smell warm earth and clover while I watch my mares nuzzle their new foals. ∎

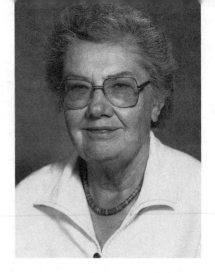

Maxine Benjamin

MAXINE BENJAMIN became one of the leading clinical pathologists of her time when her classroom notes grew into a book that became the primary text for veterinary students, animal technicians, and veterinary practitioners around the world. Published in 1958, 1961, and 1978 in English, Spanish, and Japanese, *An Outline of Veterinary Clinical Pathology* closed the ignorance gap in the use of laboratory tests to aid in the diagnosis of animal diseases. "No matter where I go in this world," says Benjamin, "people say, 'Oh, you're the one who wrote the green book.'"

Graduating in 1948 from the College of Veterinary Medicine at Colorado State University, Benjamin became assistant professor of veterinary clinical pathology at the university. In 1953 she earned her master's degree with research on shipping fever in cattle. By 1960 she was one of the first female veterinarians in the United States to become a full professor.

Benjamin was chosen as one of two Top Profs at Colorado State University in 1966. Teaching honors continued: Outstanding Educator of America in 1972, the Oliver Pennock Award for Outstanding Teaching in 1975, and the

Norden Award for distinguished teaching in the field of veterinary medicine in 1977. Benjamin also received recognition in areas other than teaching: Outstanding Woman Veterinarian in 1972; Who's Who in the West, Who's Who of American Women, and World's Who's Who of Women (1974–1975); American Men of Science, and Community Leaders and Noteworthy Americans (1975–1976); Notable Americans (1976–1977); Gaines Dog Research Center Fido Award, Colorado Veterinary Medical Association Veterinarian of the Year, and American Animal Hospital Association Veterinarian of the Year (1978).

A teacher for thirty years, Benjamin possessed a special talent to guide a developing mind from the known through the unknown to the light of discovery. An advocate of self-determination, she taught her veterinary students to believe in themselves. "From my experience," she says, "once a student has a goal, the going gets easier. It's while students flounder about, trying to find where they belong, that they have problems. Young people like to take chances because they are unaware of the obstacles, and in their brashness they often succeed."

Able to interpret a broad range of laboratory tests for the veterinary practitioner, Benjamin became a popular speaker at veterinary seminars, sometimes presenting as many as six lectures in a year. Flying from California to Florida and states in between, she stretched the boundaries of her classroom to enlighten her profession.

Benjamin retired eagerly in 1978, with no regrets and with an enormous backlog of plans. She stayed away from the university to allow new teachers—four now occupy her space—to make plans without "Max" looking over their shoulder. Now professor emeritus, Benjamin, with her wry sense of humor, describes a professor emeritus as "a person known as 'who's who' while working but upon retirement becomes 'who's that?' "

In 1987 Benjamin stepped out of retirement to teach one year at the veterinary college on St. Kitts in the Caribbean. "There, with a class of twenty-eight freshmen, I did some of my best teaching," she says.

Maxine Benjamin worked with the pioneers who brought veterinary clinical pathology to the age of sophistication. As a veterinary scientist, a teacher, and a woman, she made an indelible mark in her field. "A lot of women my age say they don't believe in women's lib, because they never needed it," she says. "I didn't need somebody to fight battles for me. I fought them for myself."

■

I was very lucky to choose a career that suited me so well. I loved clinical pathology, teaching, and the students.

I was the youngest of three children, born two years apart, but I never knew my middle brother, who was killed by a truck before I was born. My older brother was drafted in World War II and was killed as a bomber pilot. When I was four, my father died, and my mother, my brother, and I moved from Cleveland to Los Angeles to be with Mother's family.

I was a city girl, and sports ruled my life—baseball, tennis, anything that was available. I joined church just to play on their basketball and volleyball teams. Baseball was my favorite, and for a long while my pitching arm was superior to my grades as a student.

Mother and I struggled through the Depression, so there was no money put aside for college. Mother tried to guide me from her own experience and thought I should go to secretarial school. I think parents commonly underestimate the abilities of their children.

At seventeen, I attended a junior college in Los Angeles.

For twenty-five cents an hour I took whatever jobs were available—
waiting tables in a tearoom, cleaning houses, even working in a
meat-packing plant. There I took trays to the killing floor and
collected all the endocrine glands, such as pancreas, thyroid,
adrenal, pituitary. These glands were trimmed, preserved in acetone,
and later processed to extract hormones for medicine.

A chauvinistic man in the packing plant laboratory liked to
heckle the women by spraying ethyl chloride on them or in their
chair seats. Ethyl chloride gives the skin an uncomfortable burning
sensation. After cooling my fanny once too often in the meat cooler,
I suggested he lay off the spray. I had a bread pan full of defrosting
pituitaries that was filling with blood and juice. "If you spray me
once more, I'm going to throw this at you," I warned.

He persisted, and I picked up the pan. He ran for the door
as I heaved the pan halfway across the courtyard. My well-
developed pitching arm landed a perfect strike, square in his back.
The shift had changed, and the courtyard platform was crowded
with workers. There was a roar of laughter, and I got canned.
Without a job, I had to eat lightly for a month, but it was worth it.

Liking biology better than humanities, I chose a prenursing
curriculum. It took me four years to earn a two-year associate of
arts degree because I worked nights for the U.S. Corps of Engineers
in the photogrammetry section. I made maps from aerial
photographs, a skill I taught myself when my older brother gave me
a drafting set.

A woman M.D. with insufferable arrogance taught my
anatomy class at Los Angeles City College. I began to realize that
if I became a nurse, doctors like her could supervise me. Although
I didn't think so at the time, I'm indebted to her for changing my
career.

Medical school was too expensive, but after I talked to a
friend in veterinary school at Colorado State, the idea of working
with animals appealed to me. Dogs and other pets had always been
a natural part of my family.

When I applied to Colorado State veterinary college (then
called Colorado A&M), my timing was perfect. In 1944 most young
men, like my brother, were at war, and the veterinary college
accepted five women, including me, for a class that would combine
with other groups to eventually graduate thirty-two. I have always
believed that lives are governed by a matter of timing. Before the
war, very few women were accepted, and after 1948, doors at most
veterinary schools again closed to women because war veterans

had priority admission.

In my day, women veterinary students were an anomaly, and our rights were challenged all the time. We were not allowed to ride on farm calls or learn livestock reproduction skills like artificial insemination. Only a retired army colonel was tolerant enough to include women on field trips, so we traveled to dairies and packing plants.

If I had been unable to get into veterinary school, I probably would have become a medical technologist. The medical sciences are interrelated, and it's easy to jump from one to the other. I always told my students it was never too late to change if they were convinced they'd chosen the wrong career. Change was better than an unhappy lifetime in the wrong career.

During my first year in veterinary school, I waited tables in the dormitory. Starting with my second year, the dean of women took pity on me and gave me an easy job as student nurse for the dormitory. In my junior and senior years, an honor scholarship paid my tuition. I started veterinary school with six hundred dollars, and when I finished, I had three hundred. The three hundred dollars was an honorarium from the Borden Award. I won this my senior year as the student with the highest grade point average for the first three years. I was so academically oriented that setting up a practice never appealed to me.

When I first came to Colorado, I thought California was the only place to live. However, each year when I returned to Los Angeles, I found some unpleasant big-city change. When I was offered a position on the Colorado faculty after graduation, I didn't hesitate to stay in Colorado.

At first I was about the same age as my students. I had just been their cohort, so they continued to call me Max. I still lived on campus, so I ate in the cafeteria with my students. I never felt that being on the faculty made any difference. After all, I was only one grade ahead. Another faculty member overheard a student call me Max and berated the student for not using my title, "Dr. Benjamin." Professionally and socially I rarely referred to myself as "Doctor." I felt I'd achieved full status when people stopped calling me a woman veterinarian and saw me as a veterinarian.

I taught clinical pathology and one section of microbiology, supervised the diagnostic lab, and saved 25 percent of my time for my master's research. This involved the study of blood changes related to shipping fever in cattle. [Shipping fever is a pneumonia caused by one of several respiratory viruses and a *Pasteurella* bacteria and is possibly brought on by the stress of shipping and the exposure to other cattle.] Because the disease is more prevalent in winter, I remember many snowy drives to the huge Monfort stockyards at Greeley, Colorado, where I spent the morning collecting blood samples from both sick and normal beef cattle. Back then, muscular men chased the wild range animals into chutes, and all I had to do was hold the blood tubes. Even so, I lost a front tooth when a chute handle hit me in the mouth. For a while a gold tooth commemorated my master's research, but that's been replaced.

Class size and my work load at the diagnostic lab increased until the administration hired a full-time person to run the lab and gave me the choice of teaching either clinical pathology or microbiology. I chose clinical pathology and never regretted it.

No one was particularly interested in mycology [the study of fungi]. Virology and immunology were more exciting. Of course, Colorado weather was so dry that we rarely saw ringworm or other skin fungi. We saw diseases caused by systemic fungi, like blastomycosis, only in animals that came from warm, humid areas. In 1958 I went to the Centers for Disease Control in Atlanta and took its excellent course on veterinary mycology. When I returned to Colorado, I developed mycology into a postgraduate course. Fungal diseases are important because many are transmitted to humans. The trick to diagnosing fungal disease is simply to consider the possibility that it might exist. I taught a course on mycology in Africa. There fungal disease is very common in both livestock and people.

Through the years my main emphasis was always on teaching. As research became more complicated and I would have to sacrifice lab animals, my interest waned. Most of my research was limited to survival experiments at the Collaborative Radiological Health Lab in Fort Collins at the veterinary college foothills campus. The public health service funded a colony of about two thousand beagles to study the effects of low-level radiation. I was director of the clinical pathology section for three years and used automated blood-chemistry instruments to profile the large number of blood samples. We recorded normal values for dogs from birth to three years of age. This project continued almost twenty years after I left. Their great discovery was that low-level radiation did increase the incidence of cancer. When this information was transposed to humans, it was responsible, among other things, for having fluoroscopy machines removed from shoe stores.

My main objective as a teacher was to teach my students to

think. I wanted a student to come out of my exam and say, "I really had to think about that." When I was a student, I was expected to memorize, and all my thinking was done for me. For a year or so, I thought this must be the way to teach. Finally I had too much information to present in too little time. I mimeographed a detailed set of classroom notes so a student's learning wasn't based on how well he or she took notes. I taught the basics, then allowed time to discuss clinic cases in detail and demonstrate how to apply lab tests.

I used my photography skills to create a slide show of case histories. While students observed animal images, I discussed medical history, results of physical exams, and laboratory results. Like Sherlock Holmes, I led them through the case step-by-step until we discovered the diagnosis. Then I proved that the diagnosis was correct by showing pictures of the necropsy. In this way I tried to tie laboratory tests into the whole disease process and develop the student's deductive reasoning.

Over the years, I compiled thousands of case histories. I wanted to teach students that they could solve a baffling case by looking for an association with familiar signs and test results. I was not a spellbinding speaker, but when I hid behind the projector, the slides made my subject come to life.

On clinical pathology rotation, I taught either eight junior or eight senior students. I often took this small group to the university clinics to examine the animals.

When I began teaching, little was known about fluid therapy. At Colorado State we made our own solutions. Practitioners used mostly saline or dextrose and in their ignorance sometimes gave hypertonic dextrose under the skin instead of in a vein. Veterinarians also had a poor understanding about the effects of potassium and other minerals. To teach my students, I put together a series of lectures on the uses and abuses of fluid and electrolyte therapy. Practitioners were also anxious for new information, and my topic became popular at veterinary conventions. It was a situation in which, in the land of the blind, the one-eyed woman was queen.

When I was a teacher, my students researched me in advance and came prepared to deal.

"I understand you enforce the college dress code," a young man said.

"That's right," I told him.

"How do you do that?" he wondered.

"No tie, no test," I answered.

My students were always well dressed.

In thirty years of teaching I failed three students, but I managed to scare many into passing. My standards were unyielding. Students had to earn a 70 average on my exams to pass. Once, after I handed out tests, a student complained that I didn't know how to grade. "You give case histories with several parts to the question," he wrote. "I answer many parts correctly but, if I miss the diagnosis, you grade my entire answer wrong." He felt I should quit teaching.

For the final exam the student appeared, gray in complexion, and sat hunched over his test half an hour before he told me he was sick. The only place I could find for him to lie was my office floor. I noticed his membranes looked very pale. "Do you mind if I take a little blood from you?" I asked. He said he didn't. I ran a hematocrit and made a smear. His packed cell volume (PCV) was 30 percent [a very low red-blood-cell reading].

"When you tested your blood in class a few weeks ago, do you remember your PCV?"

"Forty-five percent," he said and confessed that his stools had been dark lately.

"We have to get you to your doctor," I told him.

While waiting in the emergency room, I asked him, "Do you see the importance of a correct diagnosis? If you are at a farm with a head full of facts but the farmer's cow dies because you miss the diagnosis, that farmer would not be happy."

Shortly the student was in the hospital, diagnosed as having hemorrhagic gastritis.

I taught students to milk all the information possible out of basic laboratory tests like the simple hematocrit tube before turning to exotic tests like xylose absorption. Today, instead of performing their own tests, practitioners send most samples to a commercial laboratory. There is a wait for results, and the laboratory staff interpret these results based entirely on the veterinarian's observations. Still, the foundation of an accurate diagnosis is the physical examination. Practitioners must put their hands on the animal and develop educated fingers. Lab values are used only to confirm what they see and feel.

Today's graduates are overeducated in sophisticated technology and undereducated in the basics. Before they are really competent in practice, they need more experience with animals in internships and residencies, or under the supervision of a competent, caring practitioner.

In 1967, while on sabbatical leave, I taught clinical pathology to students at New York State Veterinary School, Cornell University, Ithaca, New York. Easterners are supposed to be aloof and difficult to know, but I found the students at Cornell more open than my students at Colorado. Too quickly I discounted my department head's warning that these students might push me for concessions. My Saturday morning class had several Jewish students.

"I can't take exams on Saturday," one student told me. "It's against my religion to write."

"Well, you can talk, can't you?" I asked.

He stared at me.

"Tell me the answers," I suggested, "and I'll write them for you on the exam."

I taught from January to June and rented a country house on four acres with a swimming pool. It was always cloudy and too cold to swim. When blue sky appeared briefly, the students hollered so I could look. The entire staff of the veterinary college adopted me. They took me on hikes and loaded me with presents when I left.

In 1968 and 1969 I spent three months each year at the University of Nairobi in Kenya, organizing its laboratory and teaching clinical pathology and mycology to African students. These students were not as well prepared as U.S. students, but after four years they graduated with a bachelor of veterinary medicine degree. Most graduates worked for the government, monitoring disease and dipping livestock. Nomadic tribes, like the Masai, owned most of the livestock. I had friends at the university with camping equipment, so we went into the bush every weekend.

In 1973 I lectured at the University of Pretoria in South Africa and found a wonderful place to observe birds. Even at this time, many species of birds and animals were endangered. Agriculture was constantly encroaching on their territory. The average African family had eight children, and I saw overpopulation rapidly using up all the resources. Animals have as much right to survive as we do. In some locations they should have more rights. Man could survive without wild animals, but it would be dismal. Every time a species becomes extinct, people lose a little of their faculty to survive. In Africa and other developing countries, my experiences did not have to be pleasant to be interesting.

In 1974 I spent a month at the San Diego Zoo working with a friend who was a pathologist. Whenever any animal was handled for whatever reason, we'd draw a blood sample. In this way we established the baseline blood data for many different species. Now there is a central repository of hematological data derived from many zoos. As I look back, I realize I learned a great deal studying the blood-lymphatic system. Hematology was my favorite subject.

One of our graduates from Colorado accepted a position in the veterinary school at Ames, Iowa. She showed my classroom teaching notes to Dr. Margaret Sloss, who was a professor of clinical pathology. Dr. Sloss had lunch with people from Iowa State University Press and suggested they publish my notes. That's how my little green book, *An Outline of Veterinary Clinical Pathology*, was conceived.

Of course, I had to embellish my notes to make a book, but it was cheaper to print the books than it was for me to mimeograph my notes. The book never brought me as much fame in my hometown as it did other places. Well over fifty thousand copies sold. The final update was published in 1978, the year I retired.

I was employed from the age of seventeen and had to arrange my life around my work. I put aside many things I wanted to do and always looked forward to retirement. When I was fifty-five, I began having severe chest pains, and my physician treated me for angina pectoris. Standing while I taught seemed to encourage these pains, and I believed my life would be short.

By 1977 I was teaching 100 students, and it was difficult to keep personal contact. I wanted to know each student by name and always handed tests back on an individual basis. When I heard my class would increase to 139, I freaked out. The next year, I retired.

Without the stress of teaching, I still had chest pains so I visited a cardiologist. He listened to my heart then gave me a treadmill test.

"Well," he told me afterwards, "I don't know what's causing your pain, but it is not your heart."

I took a new lease on life. Now the pain disappears with ibuprofen.

I remember my early students best. Classes were smaller, and I met these students more often at veterinary conventions. Both Linda Merry and Jessica Porter [included in this book] were my students.

During much of my career I was the only teacher in clinical pathology. Then the college started systems that fragmented clinical pathology into areas like kidney, liver, cardiovascular, and hemic-lymphatic with a panel of teachers in each of these specialties.

After nine years in retirement, one of my friends, who was dean of the veterinary school on the Caribbean island of St. Kitts, asked me to teach clinical pathology and biochemistry. I had to work hard to update myself on new material, especially in biochemistry. I taught the biochemistry as clinical biochemistry and made a package out of each organ system. My small classes, ranging from twenty-five to forty-five first-semester freshmen, were taking anatomy, physiology, and histology concurrently, so I gave them just the background they needed to understand the laboratory tests. It was exciting to work with pliable young minds not yet cluttered with extraneous facts. I think I did my very best teaching on St. Kitts. Those students could interpret biochemical profiles better than any of my former students.

Ross University on St. Kitts is a private veterinary school designed for students who cannot get into crowded U.S. schools. In an accelerated program, students receive three years of training in two years and usually take their clinic training at Oklahoma State University, at the University of Toronto in Ontario, and at a preceptorship [apprenticeship in a practice] of their choosing. The school has a veterinary teaching hospital, but the island's main industry is sugarcane production, and animal patients are scarce.

On St. Kitts, students still groaned that my tests were too hard. After handing back the exams, I reviewed all the test questions and showed them the answers, but I couldn't convince them they should be more thoroughly prepared. Finally I played a portion of Bill Cosby's routine on "brain-damaged children."

"Now," I told them, "if you still don't know the answers, you must be brain-damaged. And I must be brain-damaged too for being here."

The grumbling stopped.

I shared a big island house with another teacher. It had a huge yard surrounded by an eight-foot wall, which protected us from the sea. Our veranda overlooked a rookery with egrets and pelicans. St. Kitts is in the Leeward group of islands about sixty miles south of St. Martin and was unspoiled by tourists. I enjoyed snorkeling in the reef just off the coast. In early spring a bad storm washed out one of the generators, and electricity had to be rationed throughout the island. I tried to schedule lectures when we had electricity. Still, there were times when my only power was my flashlight, focused on the microscope mirror. In the tropical heat our electric fans were more sorely missed than television.

Everyone should have a relaxing outlet from their daily work. I like betting games where my brain is a deciding factor. I used to play twenty-one in Las Vegas, but when they changed to multiple decks in a shoe, I lost all interest. My great love has always been horse racing. I reserved a box at Denver's Centennial horse track until it closed a few years ago. Now greyhound racing is the only game in town, and by satellite I can see the races year-round, but it does not have the same appeal as the horses.

At the Centennial I carried a folder with five-by-eight-inch cards bearing the racing-form history of every horse at the track. My game was handicapping, so I could never have too much basic information. It was great sport to match wits with the trainer and the track, trying to discover a pattern that showed a horse was reaching its peak. At big tracks I paid attention to the betting ratio between win and show. This theory says that the betting public will place money evenly on win, place, and show. The insiders, from the stables, bet only to win or place. The higher the ratio between the win and show pools, the more inside money on a particular horse. If the ratio changes in the last two minutes, it makes a horse look like a hot prospect. I always thought that picking the winner was very similar to discovering the right diagnosis in clinical pathology. Financially I probably broke even. That's not bad for entertainment.

In retirement I do things at my own pace. In 1979 I traveled to the South Pacific to meet a friend who was lecturing in Australia for three months. I stopped in Tahiti on the way to Australia, and on the way home I saw New Zealand and Fiji. The animals and birds of Australia are magnificent. I held a koala that was surprisingly heavy, like a lump of lead. Every little township in Australia and New Zealand had a racetrack. The people loved horses. In Auckland, New Zealand, I witnessed a soul-stirring race. A mare named La Mer was favored to win. She was so beautiful that I bet on her. She was last entering the stretch but lengthened her stride and thundered past the other horses for a thrilling victory.

The students and faculty of Purdue University selected me as an Old Master in 1978. Many interesting people were chosen: Father Bruce Ritter, who runs Covenant House in New York City for runaways; the female assistant attorney general from Iowa; the black female vice-chancellor and psychologist at the University of Chicago; a medical doctor from the Indianapolis Medical School; the assistant director of NASA in Houston; an entomologist from Notre Dame; Bruce Johnston, the composer who wrote "I Write the Songs"; and T. R. Ryan, the "Tumbleweed" cartoonist.

At an evening program, each of us had to speak for fifteen minutes, with no advance notice, on the personal qualities necessary in our career. I said something about independence and thinking for oneself. The next day, I met with veterinary students and faculty in a counseling session. I found three days of constant meetings very taxing but also deeply satisfying because the students showed such genuine interest. On our final afternoon all the Old Masters mingled with each other at the lovely home of the administrator, while Bruce Johnston played his songs on the grand piano. It was fun to be among such dynamic people.

I have always liked working with wood. As little as a knife and a block of wood are required to whittle a bird. One can invest thousands of dollars in woodworking equipment, but I carve with a few knives and a few gouges and burn in the feathers. If the bird turns out well, I give it away. All I invest is time and Band-Aids. I'm not creative, so there's no brain drain. Creative people think up original carvings. I simply follow diagrams and pictures.

My house is on two-thirds of an acre across from the university. I have an enormous vegetable garden. Every day I rush outside to see how many plants have emerged. My mother lived with me the last five years of her life. Now I live alone with my dog, Tinker, a Lhasa apso, and two noisy BeeBee parrots, Malcolm and Martha.

Without deadlines, I'm becoming a great procrastinator. Recently I understood why it takes me so long to complete projects. I called a busy friend on the faculty to ask her to outline a letter for me. While we were discussing the matter on the telephone, she turned on her computer and started the outline. Her secret was simply, "Don't put anything off." My daily lists started with the most enjoyable demands, and somehow I never reached the bottom. Since my revelation, I try to start with less palatable projects.

The clinical pathologist who was hired to replace me on my retirement is a supermom. She drives forty miles to work each way, she's a wonderful teacher and mother, she never says no to anybody, and she's beautiful and charming. To me, that's amazing. My career took all my energy.

On the whole I think veterinary medicine is about the same for men and women. However, I've never been attracted to working on a cow with dystocia [calving difficulty] in subzero weather on a barren range in Montana. This is manual labor. It only appeals to a man's macho image. A woman in large-animal practice doesn't have to be a wrestler. She can do the more sophisticated work and hire brawn. In the early days, I remember a clinician telling my department head that all veterinary students should have farm or ranch experience. "What would you have them do?" that wise man asked. "Dissect a tractor?"

As women increase in the profession, more areas will open

that haven't been explored. Women may be more oriented to humane work and rehabilitation. They will accept interesting positions that have less financial reward. Practice itself is expanding with more specialties and opportunities to consult.

Veterinarians I know with large bank accounts either inherited their money or made a lucky real estate investment. A person is not less rich if he hasn't earned a lot of money. Healthy, happy children can't be bought.

It is a joy to work in a profession where everyone is so motivated. As a group, veterinarians are very nice people because they are caring.

To have picked the ideal career for me was a stroke of luck. Modern veterinary students are better educated, have a better background, and are presented with more challenges, but I wouldn't trade places with today's teachers. I taught at a very exciting time, the best of times, when classes were small and personal. ■

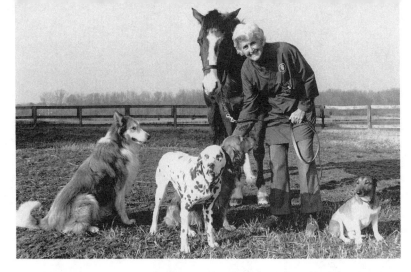

Olive Kendrick Britt

FROM HER FIRST ride at the age of three on her sorrel mule named Polly, Olive Kendrick Britt has been in the saddle—riding, training, and loving horses. Britt wanted to be a veterinarian, but in 1940 she put aside that dream to earn a bachelor of science degree in farm management from Oregon State University. "We are not always allowed to follow our first choice," she says.

For seven years Britt worked as a statistician for the U.S. Department of Agriculture. She married Ted Britt in 1941. They were divorced in late 1942 but remarried in the summer of 1943 and are still married today. Eventually Olive Britt pursued her goal of becoming a veterinarian. She received her doctor of veterinary medicine degree in 1959 from the University of Georgia at the age of forty-two. "I was lucky to be given a second chance," she says.

Upon graduation Olive Britt received the Merck Award for the greatest improvement in large-animal medicine and the A. W. Mills Award for the most proficiency in equine medicine. She is still a member of the honorary societies Phi Zeta and Phi Sigma. From 1959 to 1961 she was the first female intern-resident in the large-animal clinic

at the University of Pennsylvania's School of Veterinary Medicine. In 1961 she became the first female equine practitioner in Virginia. Britt was also the first woman on Virginia's Board of Veterinary Medicine, sitting on the board from 1978 to 1988 and serving as its president for one year. In 1983 she became an officer in the Eastern States Veterinary Medical Association, serving as president in 1989.

"I began my equine practice at the age of forty-four in central Virginia," Britt says. "I serviced ten large thoroughbred farms. Then Virginia ranked third in number of breeding farms. Now we rank fourteenth."

During twenty-nine years in equine medicine, Britt has adjusted to enormous change. She watched the opulence and grace of the large racing farms change into small estates whose residents work in Richmond. Her patients became quarter horses and Arabians kept for pleasure.

As her station wagon follows familiar bends in the road through the verdant countryside, she recalls the colorful history of many homes. The territory she covers for Virginia Equine, her employer, has grown from a radius of fifty miles to almost two hundred miles. Tall, sun-weathered, and slender, Britt is sustained by her horse work. Even in Virginia's stifling summer heat, her energy swells after each farm visit.

Now seventy-three years old, Britt walks with a slight limp and sometimes favors her left arm, in which a steel plate is screwed to the bone. (The injuries were from a car wreck, not a horse.) When she begins to talk about life as a veterinarian, the years fall from her face and she is the girl soaring over ditches on her hunter, or the auburn-haired intern showing her students how to cast the crushed carpus of a mare in foal.

"Take all the time you need to talk to Dr. Britt," said Jennifer, the wife of the owner of Virginia Equine, before the interview for this book. "She's a treasure, and it's about time somebody discovered her."

∎

I was born on a Saturday night, in London, England, during a blackout for an air raid. Mother said that as Saturday's child, I would always have to work for a living. Father was a civilian in charge of all American motor trucks sent to Russia during World War I. They were married in December of 1914, and he sailed that same afternoon for England. Mother didn't see him again until she arrived in England the next spring. I was born in 1917.

Mother tried to register my birth at the American consulate, but the people there were so curt and difficult that she registered me instead under the British flag. I had dual citizenship. At twenty-one, when I had to declare whether I wanted to be British or American, I chose American. I planned to work for the U.S. Department of Agriculture.

In 1918 my family moved to New Mexico, and Father became vice president and general manager of the second largest cattle ranch in the state, the Ladder III Ranch. It was owned by the Hermosa Land and Cattle Company, which ran 25,000 head of Hereford cattle on 500,000 acres. The ranch was in the mountains and high mesa country. I remember learning to ride in this rugged country without boundaries. The ranch still exists near Hillsboro, Sierra County, New Mexico, and several times I have returned to visit.

My sister and brother were born in New Mexico—Patricia in 1918 and William Joseph in 1922. Pat and I attended a one-room schoolhouse on the ranch. We all loved animals. I tried to ride anything I could mount, which included baby calves and Antelope, our jersey milk cow. I have a photograph of myself, barely three, sitting on Antelope and holding a chicken in my arms. My first steed was a lovely sorrel saddle mule with flaxen mane and tail.

My sister, Pat, and I were taught to care for all the animals we rode. Rusty was our sturdy burro who wouldn't move unless you sat backwards and switched his rump. Only when he turned toward home could we face forward while he ran all the way. Father gave us Ice Cream, an aged white gelding with blue eyes, and there were always chickens to chase and dogs to feed.

Mother was a strict disciplinarian, and I thank her for that now. My father often let me ride with him on the ranch. Our love for animals and the outdoors made my father and me very close.

Mother was a New Yorker and, after ten years of ranch life, finally prevailed upon my father to return to Long Island. In those days Long Island had farmland, but it was too civilized for me. When I rode in the fields and the air was clear, I could see the Chrysler Building in New York City. My father and I preferred the hardships of the ranch to the hardships of Long Island. We missed the freedom and beauty of the land.

As a civil engineer, Father started a construction business on Long Island. When the Depression began, he kept his job and made sufficient money to help Pat and me through college.

Father was an adventurer with a lust for travel. Unfortunately, he left Mother alone much of her life while he lived in many parts of the world. As he aged, he returned to New Mexico until most of his friends had died. He was retired and living in Magnolia Springs, Alabama, in 1979 when the terrible hurricane Frederick obliterated everything. When the Red Cross allowed me to find my father, I brought him to my Virginia home. A week later he died from an aneurysm.

My brother, Billy, rode as much as Pat and me, and the three of us were together most of the time. When Billy was seven, he was killed by a thoroughbred horse in a very tragic accident. Afterwards Father spoke to us: "We understand that what happened to Billy was nobody's fault, but we are going to get rid of the particular horse involved. Olive, you must decide if we should keep our other horses."

I kept the horses. Six months later, to show off to my sister, I asked my horse to jump a ditch, not knowing there was ice on the far side. My mare slipped, turned upside down, and caught me underneath. My head struck a rock. That was my first skull injury. In those days [1930], doctors weren't very knowledgeable about treating skull fractures. They prescribed rest at home. I was thirteen years old and missed that year of school.

After attending New York public schools seven years, I entered the Cathedral School of St. Mary, an Episcopal girls' preparatory school. I rode the train to school daily, and Mother gave me money to ride the bus to the station and home. Instead I saved the money and walked. Shortly before graduation, I was rich enough to buy my first English saddle and bridle.

At the end of each school year, I boarded a train to Cleveland and stayed the entire summer with my cousin Olive and her husband on their large horse farm in Gates Mills. I was named for my cousin and am a third-generation Olive. I helped exercise their hunters and polo ponies. In the heat of the summer, we rode horses early every morning and after four when it was cooler.

The awards I received in preparatory school reflect my aptitude for mathematics, my interest in language [five years each of French and Latin], and the fondness I've always felt for people. I graduated in June 1936 and had won the eighth-grade arithmetic prize, the tenth-grade prize in Latin, and the Courtesy and Fine Feeling Award. This award was a lovely leather-bound book called *The History of the Horse in Art,* which I have kept in perfect condition. I loved all sports and played on the field hockey, basketball, and lacrosse teams. I ranked second in my class, with credits in college preparatory courses, so I had no difficulty being admitted to college.

I was overwhelmed by the adjustment from my high school class of thirteen girls to a university campus. I wanted to be a veterinarian, so I entered Iowa State for preveterinary training. The veterinary faculty were not keen on women, so I quickly transferred to Ohio State where I had also been accepted. After one week on that big campus, I returned home.

I entered Adelphi College in Garden City, New York, and took science courses for one year. That summer my mother, my sister, and I took a trip west and visited colleges. I fell in love with Oregon State's campus, and its department of agriculture was friendly toward women. I decided to enroll in the College of Agriculture and had Father send my trunks to Oregon. At that time Father was ill, family funds were low, and world war threatened. I felt I should quickly complete a degree and support myself. I set aside plans to become a veterinarian and relied on animal husbandry courses to stay in contact with animals. Most of my courses were mathematics and science, and in 1940 I graduated with a B.S. in farm management. Thirteen girls started in my class, but I was the only woman to finish.

After graduation, my cousin Olive urged me to come to California and help manage her stable in Monterey. By then the Depression had robbed Olive and her husband of their Ohio farm and most of their money. Her husband was in New York starting a munitions business. During my year with Olive, she died of cancer. I closed her house and returned to Virginia.

While I was in school at Oregon, my father had bought a twenty-five-hundred-acre cattle farm in Highland County, on a ridge of the Appalachian Mountains. When I returned to Virginia, Mother was running the farm alone. Father had joined the war and was on a tugboat in the English Channel. Mother and Father had begun to live separate lives, though they remained friends.

In 1941 I married Ted Britt, whom I'd met during my year in California. In 1942 we were divorced, and we remarried in 1943. Ted was an officer in the Marine Corps, and in 1944 he sailed to Guam with the 3rd Marine Division and fought in the battle on Iwo Jima. I went to Arlington, Virginia, to live with my sister, who was working in the Civil Service Commission. With my degree and math ability, I was hired by the U.S. Department of Agriculture in their statistics and agriculture economics division. I compiled figures on crop yields and farmers' incomes. My husband and father were at war, my mother was alone on the twenty-five-hundred-acre farm, and I was unhappy.

When Ted returned unhurt, we leased seventeen acres in northern Virginia. I surrounded myself with animals. I raised as many as twenty-five hundred pheasants at one time and sold them to specialty food stores in Washington, D.C. Pheasants are incredibly dumb. They take twenty-eight days to hatch at hover temperatures of ninety-six degrees Fahrenheit, and the new chicks try to eat each other alive. I had to use a red light and red goo on the chicks to stop the pecking. I also raised broiler chickens—Rhode Island Reds and New Hampshires—and sold them at work for spending money. We kept guinea hens for their eggs, and I must say these birds were smarter than I.

My husband, I, and a retired farmer did all the work without modern farm equipment. After a while this grew tiresome. Caring for the birds did not satisfy my longing to be a veterinarian. Finally a psychiatrist told me, "Olive, you won't be happy until you do what you really want to do." I knew he was right. Ted encouraged me to return to school and become a veterinarian. The day I returned to school was the day I stopped complaining to doctors about various aches and pains.

I applied to three veterinary schools, and the University of Georgia said that when I completed the necessary science courses, it would take me. At that time [1953], Georgia had a pact with the surrounding states, including Virginia, to accept a quota of students from each state without charging out-of-state tuition. I worked half days and attended school afternoons and nights. I took organic chemistry at the University of Maryland and physics and other science courses at George Washington University. In two years I caught up and stood with the group of veterinary students from Virginia who wanted to attend the University of Georgia. Through the selection process, I became an alternate.

I returned to work and took more science courses at George Washington. In 1955 I was admitted to Georgia's freshman veterinary class. I was thirty-eight years old but no older than some classmates who were veterans of World War II and Korea. One man had been a captain and served twelve years in the Army. Our class was unusual, two women and fifty-six men of all ages who got along well. The people of Georgia were so gracious that I was not aware of any prejudice toward women at the college or on the farms.

Because of my age the dean often asked, "Olive, are you tired?" I'd say, "Tired! I haven't done anything. Why would I be tired? I'm used to working."

Since early childhood I had wanted to care for large animals, especially horses. In the veterinary clinics at Georgia, students did the castrations, delivered the calves, and examined the animals on farm calls while the clinicians supervised. Farmers never thought about suing. Today liability limits a student's hands-on experience. The clinicians do all the medical work. Students know their medicine well, but they still have to learn how to handle the livestock. Before new graduates can manage a case with authority, they need this experience to build their confidence. When I graduated in 1959, I had enough practical experience to start my own business. Still, I did not have the knowledge to be a good equine practitioner.

In the late fifties the veterinary school at the University of Pennsylvania started a two-year internship and residency program in large-animal medicine. Each year only one D.V.M. was accepted. In the class ahead of me, my friend had been chosen, and he was just finishing the program. A Harvard graduate before Georgia, he called me from Pennsylvania and told me in perfect Oxford English,

"Olive, I think it's time a woman comes into this clinic, and I've approached Dr. Raker, the head of large-animal surgery, on this. He has agreed to interview you. You are the one who ought to break the ice for women."

Dr. Charles Raker interviewed me over the Christmas holidays. "I'd love to have you," he told me, "but it's going to be a whale of a battle with the board of regents. I must get them used to the idea that a woman can do what I think you can do. If I win, you'll know by March."

Above all else, I wanted that internship. Yet, with the competition, it seemed impossible that I would be chosen. If I didn't get the internship, I needed a backup plan for after graduation.

Two internships in laboratory-animal medicine were offered by Bowman Grey School of Medicine in North Carolina, and Dr. E. W. Causey, professor of small-animal medicine at Georgia, wanted to submit my name. I would manage rats, mice, and guinea pigs in the vivarium for seventy-five hundred dollars a year, tax-free. In 1959 that was big money. Reluctantly, I let Dr. Causey send in my name.

The day I had to decide if I wanted the internship at the vivarium, I received a letter from Dr. Raker. I carried the unopened envelope in my pocket a long while before I found courage to face its contents. The first sentence is all I read: "You have been accepted as our first woman intern in the large-animal clinic and are to report July 1."

I was so excited I raced upstairs to Dr. Causey's office. "I've got it! I've got it! I'm going to Pennsylvania."

He looked so downfallen that he surprised me. "Olive, please reconsider," he said. "If not the vivarium, at least small-animal practice. You get along so well with people, and the animals love you. You're not going to earn any money as an intern."

"Don't you understand?" I responded. "The money isn't important. This is what I want to do."

At Pennsylvania, under Dr. Raker, the friendships I formed and the knowledge I absorbed created two wonderful years in my life. Although I had many fine teachers, Dr. Charles W. Raker, D.V.M., is the man most responsible for my success. He fashioned in me the knowledge and confidence to become an accomplished equine practitioner.

The head of large-animal surgery and medicine at the University of Pennsylvania's School of Veterinary Medicine for more than thirty years, Dr. Raker was at all times available to his students. Even after they graduated, he considered them members of his team. A brilliant, strong leader, he used his abilities in such a gentle, gracious manner that he coaxed from his students their best efforts. He taught me how to talk to clients to lessen their distress and not to offend. He taught me honesty. "When you lack an answer," he said, "tell people you don't know but that you'll make every effort to find out." Old enough to appreciate an adroit teacher, I was enlightened.

The veterinary buildings at the University of Pennsylvania were very old and located in the center of Philadelphia. While I was there, we cared for many of the city dray horses. At the clinic, I supervised student surgery and student treatment and medication. We were learning together, and there was enough work to give all of us unlimited experience. In addition to students, I had my caseload. Some male clients had not learned that women could work on horses. I tried to be very gracious to these men and not push them to accept me. I asked Dr. Raker not to talk clients into accepting me, but on occasion he did.

The Amish in particular did not favor a woman working on their horses. I had no wish to challenge this view, which was based on their religion. I still remember an Amish man whose horse needed a posterior digital neurectomy [delicate surgery in which the nerve supplying sensation to the posterior aspect of the foot is severed to relieve pain and lameness]. Dr. Raker insisted that I do the surgery. The Amish man stood first on one foot, then the other, and I watched his little goatee jerk up and down.

This is going to be wild, I thought. "Please," I told Dr. Raker, "this is a lot of pressure. Let someone else take the case."

We were talking practically under the nose of our client. "Olive, you do a beautiful job," he said. "These people have to realize that they are not to look at you as a woman but as a veterinary surgeon. If he doesn't want you to do it, he can take his horse somewhere else."

"You're the boss," I said, "but that's sure not what I would do."

In those days the surgery area wasn't as carefully restricted as it is now, and owners could watch from a proper distance. The Amish man refused to watch and stepped outside. I did the surgery with his horse standing in a special restraining stall. We kept the animal two or three days to be sure he healed properly. When the Amish man picked up his horse, he thanked me with a sheepish grin.

There was a tough, thickset fellow who trained standardbreds, and I asked Dr. Raker to please let me handle him my way. On several occasions while I did surgery on someone else's horse, this rough fellow watched. One day he brought a lame standardbred with a carpal fracture and pointed to me. "That's who I want to do the surgery," he said.

Dr. Raker almost fainted. I did the surgery, and after that my rough friend would accept no one else. He lived on the coast, and when he came, he always brought me a big bag of raw oysters. I shared generously with the students and staff. We were all poor as church mice, so we looked forward to such gifts.

By the time I left Pennsylvania, my ability as an equine practitioner had improved. My friend Taylor Rowe, a small-animal practitioner in Virginia, invited me to his clinic. He planned a luncheon to introduce me to all the influential horse people. Those wonderful people invited me to practice in central Virginia. Deep down I felt I owed Virginia for paying my out-of-state tuition to Georgia. I also thought it would be difficult to find suitable work with a male practitioner. It was the right time for me to open a solo practice.

I located my practice west of Richmond in Goochland County. In this area, women managed many of the small farms. These women were intrigued by a woman veterinarian, but they expected the same high-level performance from me that they consistently gave. We worked well together, and some are still close friends.

Many of the farms with horses also had cattle, Angus and Herefords. I provided routine care for the cattle, handling dystocias [difficult calving] and milk fevers. I saw some of the first Charolais, robust broad-bodied cattle from France. One farmer thought he could restrain them in a standard cattle chute. The Charolais took one big breath, and the chute fell apart. After a few years, I concentrated only on horses.

My only competitor was an older man who had successfully discouraged many male veterinarians from practicing in his area. Before I came, I wrote a letter telling him about my plans and met him in person to show him every courtesy. He told other people he didn't want me in his territory, but he never opposed me directly. Later I heard he was sick and working less. He even told some of his clients to call me. He was very prideful, but I think he felt better about me assuming his duties than a man. I practiced only a short while before he died.

I serviced ten large farms that bred thoroughbreds and maintained top racetrack stock. Under the direction of the farm manager, I often spent an entire morning on one farm, worming sixty head of horses. All of these farms were in a fifty-mile driving radius, which saved considerable time and car trouble.

I worked eight years alone before I formed a partnership with Dr. M. D. Kingsbury. We renovated a barn to serve as a clinic and built an equine practice that employed as many as five veterinarians.

I outlasted the big farms. Some owners died, and others moved to states that offered better money incentives for racetrack breeders. Their estates were subdivided, and the land is now owned by wealthy doctors and lawyers from Richmond who keep hobby farms. My practice has almost changed to a pet-horse practice. I drive many more miles in a day to treat only a few horses at each stop. Some owners understand the needs of their horses; others know nothing.

The cost of my liability insurance as an equine practitioner continues to increase. Now I'm responsible not only for the horse's welfare but also for the safety of everyone present, even the owner's children. I'm constantly filling out legal forms and writing detailed medical records on my patients.

In all these years that I have been so closely associated with horses, I have never feared them. I know their behavior, and the few serious injuries I've had have always been the result of foolishness on my part or the owner's lack of attention or understanding.

In 1975 I was called to examine some scratches on a horse's hind leg. The woman owner knew very little about horses. I told her, "Please stay on the same side with me as you hold the horse. If something happens, you can pull the horse toward us, and his back end will swing away from me." While I was examining the leg, the woman moved to the other side and pulled the horse into me. Before I knew what happened, the horse cow-kicked and knocked me down under him. My hair had just been styled, and when I fell, my head landed in a mud puddle. The rescue squad took me to the hospital, where the doctors discovered my sphenoid bone was fractured, and spinal fluid had leaked out. I was out of work several months.

Another time, I was called to castrate a horse with a nasty temperament. We didn't have effective sedation like Rompun so I tranquilized him with Acepromazine. Tap water would have been just as effective. The horse broke away from the groom and tore around the barn, finally making a sudden turn into a stall where he upended himself. The groom rushed in, and I yelled, "Keep his head down, and I'll get the casting harness." I was really very kind to that horse. I tied him tightly in the casting harness, rolled him onto his back, and scrubbed and prepared him properly for surgery.

When I began the castration, Dr. James Marshall, a medical doctor and a friend, was holding the horse's head with the nose turned up and with his weight on the horse's poll. In this position the horse could not struggle. I removed one testicle and raised my scalpel for a second incision when the horse found just enough play in the rope around his hock to knock my elbow. The scalpel blade was driven deep into my left palm, severing nerves and tendons.

Dr. Marshall was horrified. "Olive! You've got to stop. You're bleeding and have a dreadful injury."

"Hold on to his head, please! You know I can't stop now."

"You can't finish," he said.

"I'm going to finish. If you don't stay on his head, everything will be lost."

I finished, mostly one-handed, and further damaged my injured hand by stretching the cut tendons. I was worried the horse would bleed to death or something equally terrible, but he healed later with no trouble.

As soon as I finished, Dr. Marshall gave the horse to a groom and wrapped a sterile towel around my hand. "Olive, I'm taking you to the hospital," he said. "You've done some major damage."

"No," I told him, "I'm full of blood, and I'm going home first to change clothes."

When I arrived home, my brother-in-law was there and insisted that I let him drive me to the hospital. Dr. Marshall had called him, as well as the leading hand surgeon in Richmond, who was waiting for me at the hospital. In surgery I requested a local anesthetic and the surgeon worked two hours to pull that mess together.

"You don't want to watch," he told me.

"Yes, I do," I said. "I want to see if you're doing a good job." I'm sure he thought I was crazy.

I was out of work for a while, going to therapy to return function to my fingers. There was no improvement, so I returned to work and asked a friend to be my driver. I did what I could one-handed, but without thinking I also tried to use my left hand. After a while my fingers began to function, and in three months I was doing the things I'd always done.

Before my clients purchase a horse, they often ask me to

determine the animal's fitness. As part of my examination, I used to ride the animal. Now that I'm older, I have to watch someone else ride, but I still recognize good horsemanship and its effect on a horse's gait. Horse people know me for my proficiency in lameness diagnosis and prepurchase examination.

In the summer of 1980, with a group of six I joined a float-pack trip into Montana wilderness. We camped, fished, rode horses, rafted the rapids, all the things I love to do in untamed country. After that trip I was more aware of aches and pains accumulated from various horse and car accidents. Riding was less comfortable. My last ride on a horse was in 1984, with Dr. Kingsbury, my partner in practice for fifteen years. We rode seven hours through the Blue Ridge Mountains. When I climbed down, I was stiff, but later there was no soreness, just a wonderful memory.

I returned to solo practice in 1985. A year later my life almost ended. It was dusk and raining. I was returning home from my last call, traveling forty-five miles per hour, ten miles under the limit, on a winding two-lane road. Suddenly car headlights were directly in front of me, and I couldn't turn away. That fearful, blinding light is my last memory. The crushing impact occurred in front on the driver's side. An ambulance from a nearby country store arrived, and its people gave me first aid until my county ambulance arrived. I was only semiconscious, but I wouldn't allow anyone to move me until my sister, a registered nurse, arrived. I kept asking my sister how badly my car was damaged.

"Olive, we must worry about you!" she said. "The car will be fine."

I was hospitalized three weeks. My orthopedic surgeon placed a bone plate on the fracture of my right ulna and used bone screws to repair the compression fracture near my knee in my left tibia. My left ankle was also fractured and is the reason I now limp. The badly damaged ankle joint stiffened. Fortunately the weather was cold, and my heavy coat padded my impact with the steering wheel. I suffered several broken ribs and severe contusions to one lung lobe. My teeth were damaged, and my face and head badly bruised.

The driver of the other car was unhurt. In fact he climbed out and walked home before the ambulance arrived. Later the police found him drunk in his home with a drink in his hand. According to Virginia law, if the police don't apprehend a person within ten minutes from the time of their offense, their blood alcohol level cannot be tested. This man was never convicted of drunk driving.

After many months of physical therapy, I regained the use of my arm and leg. To this day I have not seen my car and continue to avoid photographs of the accident. I was driving a Ford Ranchero with a heavy insert on the back for my medical supplies. The impact jarred the insert loose. It crashed through the rear window and completely destroyed the passenger side. My life was spared by inches.

Dr. T. J. Newton, who owned his own horse practice in the area, took over my solo practice to help me while I healed. After a year, I decided to return to work. Dr. Newton told me, "Olive, you really don't want to be by yourself in practice. Can't we work something out?"

Now I'm a contract veterinarian with Virginia Equine, owned by Dr. Newton. He includes me in many of the decisions. I returned to practice slowly at first, but now I handle a full schedule with no difficulty. I realize I'm restricted not only by my age but also by my injuries, and I'm not as prideful as I used to be.

Recently I answered a call on a mare who, the owner said, was down with colic. When I arrived, two women and the owner, an older man, drove me to the mare, way out in the field. I began my examination and immediately realized the mare did not have colic but was straining to deliver a foal. I reached into her uterus and discovered the foal was upside down with its head turned back. I had brought equipment to treat colic but did not have my obstetrical chains. Even if I'd had the proper equipment, I wasn't at all sure I had the strength to turn that foal. I sent the women to phone the closest veterinarian and ask him for his help.

While we waited, I went to work. With plastic sleeves on both arms and lubricated, I reached into that uterus up to my shoulder. Because this was the mare's first foal, her pelvis had not sprung, and there was very little space for movement. The mare's contractions squeezed my arms between the foal and the pelvis bones. Fortunately I was able to flip the baby over on the first try and straighten the head.

The owner was standing beside me. I looked him straight in the eye. "You have got to help me pull this baby out, and we can't let it drop on the ground," I said. "Can you do that?"

He assured me he could. When that strong mare contracted, we pulled the foal's legs until we delivered her baby. I sent someone back to call the other veterinarian and save him a thirty-mile drive. The maiden mare did not understand how to care for her baby, and the weather was too cold to leave them in the field. With the owner's help, I finally pushed and pulled the pair into the barn and coaxed the mare into nursing her baby.

Afterwards my arms ached and turned black and blue, but I was thankful I was able to handle that dystocia. Now I'm content to let others deliver foals. I have lost considerable physical strength, although my mind, unaffected by at least four head injuries, is as good as ever. Still, I admit my limitations, because a poor animal is relying on me and I don't want to fudge it up.

When I first started practice, I was very proficient at surgery, but I was limited because my surgery had to be done in a field. Over the years surgery became secondary. When I associated with Dr. Kingsbury, we performed complicated surgery in a barn remodeled as a modern surgical suite. Now I'm back to simple field surgery. I administer new drugs like Rompun and Ketaset and use portable gas anesthetic machines with Halothane to keep a horse sleeping as long as necessary. After gas anesthesia a horse can walk in forty-five minutes. I refer difficult surgeries to the modern large-animal hospitals only two to three hours from us.

The state of Virginia has very strict rules governing animal hospitals and vehicles driven in practice. They inspect and license our hospital and mobile units. The Virginia Board of Veterinary Medicine creates and enforces these standards. I was the first woman appointed by the governor to this board, and I served ten years, from 1978 to 1988. There were five veterinarians on the board, and the governor later appointed one citizen member. We hired inspectors to enforce our standards. These inspectors were strict but fair. In the last few years Virginia animal hospitals meet the even stricter codes set by the American Animal Hospital Association. Our board has a great deal of control, but it's all for the good. Very few veterinary hospitals or veterinarians are forced from practice. Instead the board helps them comply with the rules.

I practiced twenty-nine years in Virginia, and many of the veterinarians that the board reprimanded were my friends. It was difficult not to be partial. Many problems arose from poor communication between practitioner and client. I learned that a fair decision is not easy to make.

Over the years I have seen the science of veterinary medicine become so advanced that it replaced the art. The art of veterinary medicine is being able to use your knowledge and perform your service in a smooth, pleasant way, so you feel good about what you are doing. You and the client form a bond of true concern for the animal. Professionals who rely on scientific knowledge only become frustrated when they must deal with human emotions. I believe it is as important to like and understand the owners as it is the horse. Most good veterinarians, like any good medical person, are very happy. When young people consider veterinary medicine, they have to realize it is a lovely, fulfilling way of life, but they will not earn monumental sums of money.

As an equine practitioner, I go to the home of my patients and perform my work in front of the owner. When necessary, I try to comfort the owner. The setting is more personal than the exam room in an animal clinic. A woman may ask for me because I treated her first pony when she was a child.

I see signs that people will find less destructive ways to live and save the natural world. As people return to the land, they increase their interest in horses. In Virginia the driving horse is making a comeback, and driving clubs are forming.

Virginia is currently fighting to build a racetrack. If we get the nod, thoroughbred breeders will return. I live on ten acres that was once part of one of the largest and most famous racing farms in Virginia. Riva Ridge and Secretariat were born there. I was the farm's veterinarian for fourteen years, until it dissolved and was sold in 1979. I would love to see breeders like that return.

My marriage to Ted Britt has endured forty-six years even though, for the most part, we have kept separate homes and careers. Early on, we decided that I would pursue veterinary medicine wherever it took me, and Ted would follow engineering sales in the corporate world. We became trusting friends, always supporting each other, but we lost the close bonds of a standard marriage.

When we first met, we looked so much alike—tall, dark-haired, athletically slim—that people thought we were brother and sister. Strangely, neither of us found someone else. Now, because we are the same age, we both think about slowing down. Ted works in Washington, D.C., and we are together on weekends. Perhaps age has softened our stubborn and opposite wills, and we can live together in a more traditional marriage. Marriage is not always an easy road for professional couples.

I truly love horses and dogs and all animals. For seven years Butch, my collie, rode with me on all my calls, and everyone became his friend. How thankful I am that I was given a second chance to become a veterinarian. In this profession I've always been free to express myself. Some days I awake and have little aches and pains, but when I look out and see the morning sun, I know I'm alive and have patients waiting for me.   ■

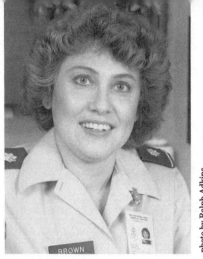

photo by Ralph Adkins

Joanne Rick Brown

IT ISN'T every woman who can do thirty push-ups, rappel off the side of a tower, radio for a medical evacuation helicopter, find her way in unknown terrain with only a map and a compass, and hit a bull's-eye with a .45 automatic or M-16 rifle, but then, Lt. Col. Joanne Rick Brown never pretended to be just like everyone else. Even in high school, when some girls her age were twirling batons and leading cheers at the pep rally, Joanne was off in some show-ring, leading her horse through its paces. In the years since high school, Joanne has never been far removed from horses— her own or those belonging to Uncle Sam. Brown's roles today are varied— Joanne, Mommy, the commander's wife, Dr. Brown, or Lt. Col. Brown—and she is just as comfortable in a riding habit, fatigues and combat boots, a cocktail dress, or a white lab coat.

A short woman with curly chestnut hair, Joanne is used to breaking ground.

Joining the army in 1972, she was the second female officer in the Veterinary Corps and, since entry, has been the ranking woman. In 1974 she commanded an all-male unit in Korea. Her vocation as an army veterinarian has taken her from the icy cold of the Arctic Circle to the dry heat of the deserts of Bahrain and many places in between.

Brown has received numerous military awards and decorations, including an Army Commendation Medal, an Expert Field Medical Badge, and two Meritorious Service Medals. She holds a master's degree in veterinary microbiology and is a member of the American College of Veterinary Preventative Medicine. Brown is now chief of the Regional Veterinary Laboratory, Walter Reed Army Medical Center, with duty at Fort Meade, Maryland.

I will always have horses. They are like family. I am down to one mare now, but she's rather special because I owned her mother and raised her myself. I got my first horse when I was twelve years old, and even when I went away to college, I managed to take two or three horses along with me. I've been traveling with horses ever since.

I decided in junior high that I would combine my love of horses with science by becoming a veterinarian. I lived at that time with my parents and three younger siblings in Crystal, Minnesota, a suburb of Minneapolis. My dad owned a sporting goods store, and my mother and grandfather were pharmacists.

My mother, who had become a pharmacist in the days when few women pursued that career field, knew that veterinary medicine would be a difficult course of study for me. At that time the University of Minnesota admitted only one or two token women into each veterinary school class, but Mother and I both had the confidence that I could make it if I was strong and persistent.

After high school graduation in 1966, I enrolled at the University of Minnesota in St. Paul. I managed to find a farm close by my sorority house for my horses. After only two years of preprofessional studies, I was accepted by the College of Veterinary Medicine at the University of Minnesota. I was nineteen years old and one of the youngest in the freshman class.

I don't recommend that anyone attempt veterinary school after only two years of preveterinary courses. I had taken only the required subjects and would have benefited from more college experience. Most students who enter veterinary schools today have B.S. degrees, and a significant number have advanced degrees.

I was one of six women and sixty men who made up the freshman veterinary school class. The years that we spent in veterinary school, 1968 to 1972, were turbulent times on college campuses. The Vietnam War, campus protests, and changes in many areas were taking place. For example, we had a strict dress code when I was a freshman. The women were required to wear dresses, except in large-animal clinics, and the men wore white shirts and ties. By the time we graduated, everyone was wearing blue jeans, and the men were beginning to appear at school with beards and mustaches.

We women students had to prove ourselves, especially in large-animal clinics. Because I am small, I sometimes had problems wrestling cows and horses. I remember one time when I was assisting with surgery on a large holstein cow with a displaced abomasum [a chamber of the stomach]. It was my duty to reach around the abomasum and bring it into position so the surgeon could suture it to the abdominal wall. I tried and tried, but I simply could not reach enough of the organ to pull it around. I also had difficulty palpating large workhorses, but I'm great at delivering baby pigs and other procedures requiring small hands and arms.

When I was a senior, I had the fantastic opportunity to spend a two-week externship in equine medicine. The first week I stayed with Dr. Bill Solomon and his family at Castleton Farms in Lexington, Kentucky. Castleton Farms, a standardbred breeding farm, was the home of Bret Handover and Good Times, two very famous standardbred stallions. While at Castleton, I examined two hundred mares by rectal palpation to determine pregnancy and the state of the reproductive organs; although the aesthetic nature of this procedure is dubious, it was a great learning experience. I would have loved a job in equine breeding-farm medicine, but openings were limited at that time for a woman with no experience or contacts.

My second week was spent with Dr. Gary Lavin, who owned the Twin Spires Veterinary Hospital at Churchill Downs. This was my first exposure to racetrack medicine. It seemed to me that racetrack veterinarians spent much of their time listening to and catering to the whims and desires of horse trainers and owners at the track. Dr. Lavin spent mornings at the track and afternoons in surgery at the hospital.

My love for horses was one of the common bonds that I shared with my two roommates, Jan and Jill. The three of us, called the Terrible Trio by our classmates, shared an apartment for three of our four years in veterinary school. We are still friends. Jan Spencer now owns a racehorse breeding ranch in Utah, and Jill McClure is a member of the veterinary school faculty at Louisiana State University, Baton Rouge. Jan and Jill married veterinarians. I dated a young man in the Army Special Forces and later married a career soldier.

Soldiering as a profession was assumed to hold no interest for women veterinarians. When the Army recruiters came to talk to my junior class, the women were excused. During my senior year, however, I stayed and inquired about assignments for veterinary officers. All officers spend a couple of weeks in the Army basic course at Fort Sam Houston in San Antonio and two months in the veterinary course in Chicago. After completion of those two courses, I could accept a two-year assignment at Fort Carson in Colorado Springs.

Fort Carson had a lot of appeal because it offered a boarding facility for privately owned horses, a stable of forty Recreational Services horses, an equine cavalry unit, the military working dogs, and an outpatient veterinary clinic. The military also sounded adventurous to me, and I was enticed by the opportunities to travel. Plus, I figured that I could stand anything for the required two years.

Dr. Jean Sessions, who had been an Army veterinarian from 1970 to 1972, was the first woman veterinary officer. She had left the army by the time I joined, so I was the second woman to become a member of the Army Veterinary Corps.

When I took the Army basic course, I was the only woman in a class of more than 250 medical officers. I found that it was impossible to be one of the boys. I tried to be myself and do everything that was expected of a military officer. Today there are 55 female officers in the Army Veterinary Corps, but in the early days, there was only me.

After veterinary school graduation and before I reported for duty with the Army, I spent a wonderful summer showing my quarter horse mare, Bar-B-Bandit. The timing was perfect for me to relinquish the showing of my horse to a trainer when I left for the Army basic course. The trainer exhibited Bar-B-Bandit in Chicago while I was stationed there and showed her in Colorado when I moved to Fort Carson. Bar-B-Bandit then found a home at the Fort

Carson boarding facility, which came under my jurisdiction.

Horses were not my only wards on base. I also handled the care of the military working dogs and ministered to the needs of pets belonging to army personnel. It was not always easy. I was very young and youthful in appearance, as well as female, and the dog handlers were embarrassed and reluctant to talk to me about the private parts of a dog. Military pet owners didn't seem to get the idea that I was a real veterinarian. I would walk into the exam room at the base veterinary clinic and introduce myself as Captain Rick. After I spent another fifteen minutes taking a medical history and examining the pet, the owner would ask me when the veterinarian would be in.

I was determined that my gender would not keep me from trying new and unique experiences. My boss at Fort Carson, Col. William Van Zytveld, knew that I had never ridden in a helicopter and would very much like to, so he arranged for me to take part in the Dust-Off exercise, designed to train medical personnel to load and secure injured patients in medical evacuation helicopters.

Much to my surprise, I learned that I was the intended patient when a voice announced over the loudspeaker, "And our patient today is Captain Joanne Rick." I finally realized that I was supposed to lie on the ground and pretend to have a broken leg. It was then that I turned to the young, good-looking operations officer who was in charge of the Dust-Off demonstration and asked him to hold my purse. The medics lifted me onto a litter and loaded me into the helicopter. We flew away and left Frank Brown "holding the bag."

Of course, I had to see Frank again to retrieve my purse, and we were soon dating seriously. Frank, who was a captain in an Air Defense artillery unit, received orders for Korea. We decided to get married before he left in March 1974.

I remember when my husband first told his colleagues that he was going to marry an Army veterinarian. One of his buddies replied, "I bet I know why Frank's going to marry her. She can probably pick him up with her left hand and throw him against the wall." When they met me, they were really surprised.

I asked for an assignment in Korea, and we were advised to marry quickly if we wanted a joint tour. The army had few married couples at that time, and married housing was nonexistent. We had to get an exception to policy to share a BOQ [bachelor officers quarters] in Korea.

I spent my first few months in Korea attached to a food

inspection unit. Then I became the commander of the 477th Medical Detachment Small Animal Hospital. I was in charge of animal care and control of animal diseases, such as rabies, which might be transmitted to people. I enjoyed my work and spent seven days a week at it. I was instrumental in getting the hospital renovated and the older sentry dogs replaced by younger dogs.

Because I was the first woman in charge of an all-male veterinary unit, my superiors kept a close eye on me to see how I performed. They must have been satisfied, because in 1983 they sent another female veterinary officer to Honduras with an all-male team. I also received the Army Commendation Medal for my service in Korea.

After Korea, Frank and I were stationed at Fort Bliss in El Paso, Texas. He finished a B.S. degree in business administration there, and I completed the Army Medical Department advanced course in San Antonio. I also earned the Expert Field Medical Badge (EFMB) while in San Antonio. Recipients of the EFMB must complete a grueling two days of written, oral, and practical tests, plus a physical fitness test, day and night map-reading courses, and a twelve-mile road march. Anyone who wears the EFMB has definitely earned it.

One of the advantages of the military is the opportunity to pursue advanced civilian education. After Frank graduated with a B.S. degree, he was assigned to the District Recruiting Command in Houston, and I started a master's degree program in veterinary microbiology at Texas A&M in College Station. Luckily, Houston and College Station are less than a hundred miles apart, because we maintained a commuter marriage for two years.

We had been promised an assignment in Germany after I graduated. As it turned out, I went to Germany first, and Frank followed seven months later. He thought it was wonderful; I already had a house and a car and everything set up when he came over.

I was stationed in Germany for four years. I spent seven months as officer-in-charge of the Food Hygiene Branch of the 64th Medical Detachment in Vogelweg and then became assistant chief and finally chief of the Division of Veterinary Medicine of the 10th Medical Laboratory in Landstuhl.

The assignment in Europe was my favorite. I traveled all the way from Norway and Iceland to Bahrain and Israel and everywhere in between to inspect dairy processing plants that sold Grade A dairy products to the military. I traveled in civilian clothes and looked just like everyone else. When I stepped out of my car or plane, I was met by military or civilian personnel who lived in the area and was provided with transportation to the local plants and sights and an interpreter, if needed. Occasionally, a middle-aged plant manager was reluctant to accept my authority because of my gender, but for the most part, I was well received and saw a side of the European and Middle Eastern culture that was closed to tourists.

When I traveled to Norway to inspect two dairy plants, I spoke to the Norwegian Army Quartermaster School in Oslo about our dairy testing program in Europe. I was also invited to lecture at the Norwegian Royal College of Veterinary Medicine about women in the U.S. Army Veterinary Corps.

I went from Oslo to north of the Arctic Circle to participate in a NATO exercise. The Norwegian Veterinary Corps was in charge of providing veterinary services for the exercise because it was held in Norway. I followed along with them to gain firsthand experience in cold-weather operations. We checked food supplies and camps to see that everything had been cleaned up and disposed of properly. Some of the units melted snow for water, and we checked it to make sure it was safe for drinking.

Toward the end of my time in Europe, I traveled to another frigid country, Iceland. My daughter, Jennifer, was four months old at the time, and I was fortunate enough to have a nanny at home who could care for her while I was gone. Iceland was my last big trip before we returned to the States.

Jennie came into Frank's and my life at a rather late date and is very important to us. She is growing up surrounded by women who are doctors, lawyers, and soldiers. I don't think it will ever occur to her that she can't do something just because she is female.

I am often called upon to give presentations about women in military veterinary medicine to veterinary college groups. I usually tell my audience that a career in the Army Veterinary Corps, like any career, has advantages and disadvantages. For me, the advantages outweigh the disadvantages, but everyone must decide that for himself or herself. I think the opportunities for travel and education are phenomenal. The competitive salary, the thirty days of paid vacation, the retirement plan, and other benefits are incentives to join. To emphasize the benefits, I usually mention that I utilized the military medical plan when I was pregnant, and my daughter cost a mere $11.56, an amount I remember because I put the receipt in Jennie's baby book.

Jennie was only eighteen months old when Frank became commander of the 2-62 Air Defense Artillery Battalion with the Light Infantry Division at Fort Ord, California. I assumed the position of operations officer for the Fort Ord Veterinary Services. Veterinary Services included six branches at other bases in California, and I traveled frequently to substitute for officers on leave or temporary duty. I was also a training officer, and one of my areas of interest was client relations.

Military people often complain about the impersonal treatment they receive at Army medical facilities. I didn't want that to happen at base veterinary clinics. I presented a seminar on effective client relations to veterinary personnel at all the Fort Ord branches. Today I give the talk to the 91Ts [animal-care specialists] at their Walter Reed school.

Understanding the client and effective communication are extremely important. We should talk with people in a courteous manner and in the kind of language they understand. I teach telephone etiquette, how to greet the client, how to handle anger and frustration, the human-animal bond, the death of a pet and stages of grieving, and the different types of pet ownership.

A large percentage of pet owners, like me, consider their pet to be part of the family. They can be extremely stressed when that animal is sick or dying and may react in what might be considered an inappropriate manner. We've all experienced the owner who is filled with guilt or remorse about the pet's illness or the owner who reacts with anger directed toward veterinary personnel. In other cases, the bond between the owner and pet is less strong—the pet may be a status symbol or the kids' pet.

More than 50 percent of the veterinary technicians in the modern Army are female. I think that women are drawn to this field because it enables them to use natural traits of nurturance and empathy. It's the same reason more women are entering veterinary school today.

One of the many roles I played at Fort Ord was that of the commander's wife. I wanted to participate in all of the activities that were expected of me, but finding the time or energy to do so was hard. Jennie was a toddler, and as always, the horses had to be fed and cleaned. Yet the opportunity to make friends and work with women was very rewarding.

One of the activities I enjoyed was family day, which was set up so that military wives could participate in the same type of training as their husbands. In one exercise, the wives rappelled off the tower, and I went first to prove that it could be done without loss of life or limb. We really felt like we had accomplished something at the end of the day, and it was one more thing that the wives could share with their husbands.

I have seen changes in the outlook and expectations of military wives. Some of the changes have been good, and some have not. The young wife of today is more independent, better educated, and more knowledgeable about the military and its way of life, and most work outside the home. Though this may be positive, many wives are no longer available for volunteer work, and numerous services of the Army community depend upon volunteer workers. Some of the young wives cannot abide the very real dedication and selflessness that it takes to pursue a career in the military. It is not easy to pick up and move your family every two to three years, live in a foreign country, or tolerate long absences of one's spouse. Some wives simply can't or won't handle these aspects of military life.

Moving to a new and sometimes exotic location can be an exciting experience or a very difficult one, depending on your outlook, your sense of adventure, your organizational skills, and the amount of junk in the attic or basement. With nine moves behind me, I can easily transport two horses, three cats, two cars, a truck and trailer, one child, and a husband across the United States without batting an eyelash.

I am currently stationed at Fort Meade, Maryland, as chief of the Regional Veterinary Laboratory at Walter Reed. Our major missions are food analysis and animal diagnostic work with an emphasis on rabies and Lyme disease.

I also serve as a consultant for the ceremonial horses stationed at Fort Myer. I was project officer for the team of horses that participated in President Bush's inaugural parade. The caisson horses, which are used to pull the caisson and coffin when there's a burial at Arlington National Cemetery, are matched teams of draft horses. I occasionally get a call to take a look at one of those big fellows.

I started with horses, and I've managed to stay with them. My ten-year-old mare is boarded twenty-seven miles away from home, but I arrange my schedule so I can ride two or three times each week. I hired a housekeeper who comes to my home eight hours each week. It's worth spending the money to make time for riding, because it is so important to me. I belong to a hunt club, and we hunt on farms that are close to where I board my horse.

I also employ a baby-sitter to care for my daughter, who is now six years old. This surrogate grandmother is the same dear woman who took care of Jennie when we were stationed here before. If I have to be on the firing range at 6 A.M., I leave my daughter at the sitter's home the night before. If Frank and I are both gone, Jennie may stay with the sitter for a week or longer.

I feel fortunate that I make an adequate salary and can afford what I consider good child care. It concerns me that so many women with small children have to work at low-paying jobs to make ends meet and that their children may be receiving inadequate care and guidance. These children are vulnerable to drugs, which have been so readily available in the D.C. area.

I don't know of any easy answers to the drug problem. The Army has taken steps to reduce substance abuse among its soldiers. I share the building with the drug testing laboratory, and drug testing is mandatory in all Army units. An officer who tests positive will be discharged, and an enlisted person who is identified as having a problem is quickly routed into a treatment program. The young troops are getting the word, because drug use is decreasing in the Army. There has also been a real push to stop the happy hour at officers clubs and NCO [noncommissioned officers] clubs. Alcohol is rarely served at military functions today.

The Army knows that, to be effective, its soldiers must be drug- and alcohol-free, as well as physically and mentally conditioned. We are required to pass a PT [physical training] test every six months. The PT test includes a two-mile run, push-ups, and sit-ups, as well as stepping on the scales. If a person strays over the weight limit, he or she is put in the weight program. It is definitely an incentive to stay in shape and requires discipline. I feel good, so I consider it a positive requirement of my job.

My job has been easier, I think, because I am married to an Army officer. Frank and I understand and support each other because we know firsthand the obligations that a career in the military demands. He has been very supportive of my career, and I try to do the same for him. I think it would have been more difficult if I was a civilian veterinarian married to a military officer. If I wanted to practice, I would have to pass a state board in each state, as well as find new employment after each move. I also think that female Army veterinarians who are married to civilian men face similar problems. It takes a special man to understand the commitment and to handle moving to new locations. Because women still assume most of the family obligations, women in the

Veterinary Corps are not staying as long as their male counterparts. After one of two assignments, they usually move into a field that will accommodate a family easier.

It would probably be helpful to women who face these unique stresses to have a good networking system. However, our numbers are still small, and we are spread too far apart to meet other women veterinarians who could serve as mentors. We rarely have the chance to work with another woman veterinarian. In most cases, the mentors have come from the male sector. Gen. Robert Jorgensen and his wife, Dorothy, certainly went out of their way to encourage me and give me advice about my military career. He is retired now, but I consider him the rock that has always been there for me.

The unsung heroes of female veterinary officers have often been the wives of senior officers who establish policy. These women work behind the scenes to support us and to run interference for us at dinner tables all over the world.

Military veterinary medicine is broader in scope than just food inspection or animal practice, and as I grow in knowledge and experience, I find my interests changing. Although I still enjoy working with animals, I am now drawn to the public health and preventative medicine aspect of our profession.

I recently developed an SOP [standing operating procedure] titled "Precautions for Pregnant Veterinary Personnel." It covers biological, radiological, chemical, and physical dangers, as well as recommendations for dealing with them. This SOP will serve as a pattern for all the military veterinary clinics and research laboratories. This sort of thing is just as exciting and satisfying as diagnosing an animal case.

Veterinary medicine is more than just a job to me—it's my life. I'm terribly proud to be a veterinarian and to work in my chosen profession. I became a veterinarian for very simple reasons—my love for animals and science—and veterinary medicine has allowed me to fulfill both of those passions. ∎

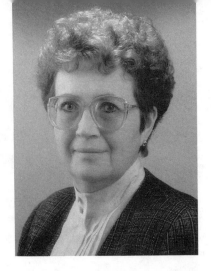

Ann Schola Clark

TRYING TO CATCH Ann Schola Clark is like trying to corner a drop of quicksilver. In 1989 Clark became the director of the Career Development Center at the American Veterinary Medical Association. That new position took advantage of her energy to set in motion a national career placement and expansion service for veterinarians. Now she is doing what she likes to do: keeping veterinarians in touch with each other. "I'm always working," she says. "I talk to a million people a day with a dozen ideas, and I'm having fun."

Clark received her doctor of veterinary medicine degree in 1964 from the College of Veterinary Medicine at Ohio State University, Columbus. While she was married to Dr. George C. Clark, a navy dentist, Ann Clark practiced small-animal medicine on the move with her husband, first in South Carolina and twice in Washington, D.C. After her two sons were born, Ann Clark worked for the Food and Drug Administration's Bureau of Veterinary Medicine in Rockville, Maryland.

In 1976 Clark was the first female veterinarian to join the staff of the American Veterinary Medical Association (AVMA) in Schaumburg, Illinois. She was hired as an assistant editor and later as an associate editor for the organization's two journals, the *American Journal of Veterinary Research* and the *Journal of the American Veterinary Medical Association (JAVMA)*. Both refereed journals, they are the sources of veterinary medical information that are quoted most often in scientific literature. Every member of the AVMA, which includes 90 percent of U.S. veterinarians, receives a copy of the semimonthly *JAVMA*.

Ann believes that her six years in practice have helped her succeed in association work. "In practice, I tested science in the real world, and I learned what made sense," she says. "This made me more effective as an editor. Most AVMA members are practitioners. Because I've been there, I know how they feel. This is important when I'm trying to develop a service they will use."

∎

From the age of five, I wanted to be a veterinarian. Nobody ever told me women couldn't be veterinarians. My mother said that *veterinarian* was the only word I ever bothered to learn to spell.

My concept of medicine came from my father, who had a bachelor of science degree in zoology and a master's in education. After my father had been accepted at the University of Pittsburgh medical school, his father died. That was during the Depression, and my father gave up going to medical school to support his family. In the end, my father owned and ran a Sohio service station in Akron, Ohio. He was my biggest supporter.

I never considered human medicine as a career, only veterinary medicine, but my father was thrilled with my choice. Unfortunately, he never saw me receive my D.V.M. degree. He died as I started my senior year in veterinary school.

As a child, I was on a different track from that of other people. I loved to spend a day alone with my boxer, Budge, which I showed at dog shows and took through obedience training. I never dragged home injured birds or stray animals. Neither my parents nor my brother, who was five years younger, were true animal lovers. Still, we always had a dog and, once, a rabbit. My mother took our dogs to a veterinarian on a regular basis.

Horseback riding was a rare treat. Once, I read how you were supposed to bridle and saddle a horse. I tied my mount to a tree and practiced until it became easy. If I felt the poor rental horse was tired, I'd dismount and walk beside him.

My mother was always available to take my brother and me anywhere we needed to go. Our life-style required transportation by car, so my mother was in perpetual motion.

I attended Garfield High School in Akron, a middle-class school where less than half the students were college-bound. Mother, educated in business school, viewed college as important for my brother and me. After I received my doctor of veterinary medicine degree, my mother thought I was the world's most brilliant surgeon and diagnostician. Yet she would worry that I'd pinch my finger in a door. I thought about asking her, "Mom, do you have any idea how dangerous my work can be?" But I really didn't want her to change.

In high school we didn't have career counselors or books on a veterinary career, so I visited Ohio State University in Columbus during my junior year for firsthand information. I was seventeen and had an appointment with Dean Russell Rebrassier. The main veterinary building with the dean's office was so old that when I tried to enter, the screen door fell off in my hand. Undaunted, I met the dean and found out what courses I would need in high school to be considered for veterinary medicine. If people said "A woman can't be a veterinarian," I didn't hear them.

In my freshman year as a preveterinary student at Ohio State University, my city background gave me considerable anxiety. If I knew nothing about livestock, I would have no credibility with livestock producers. At 8 A.M. I took a course titled "Feeds and Feeding." The instructor talked about things on a farm I'd never heard about before. At 9 A.M. I bought coffee for two classmates, while they translated what the instructor had said. They explained sorghum and millet, liming a field (somehow I knew the farmers weren't pouring on gallons of limeade), and disking or harrowing a field. Even the fact that cows had four parts to their stomach was a surprise to me.

The Saddle and Sirloin Club at the university sponsored a livestock show once a year. Students could select a university animal to work with and show. Every year I participated. After a while I could catch and halter most large animals, lead livestock in a show-ring, and recognize different animal breeds.

I took livestock production courses in poultry, sheep, swine, cattle, and horses. For one livestock show, I was assigned a Suffolk sheep and expected to prepare it for the show-ring. That one sheep taught me about sheep behavior and wool. I had to keep its wool washed, trimmed, and blocked and finally shear it.

Years later, I worked for the Food and Drug Administration and visited the research station at Beltsville, Maryland, with a group of U.S. Department of Agriculture officials. I was the only veterinarian in the group who could recognize all the breeds of sheep.

I was determined not to let any deficiency be a handicap. By weaseling my way into agronomy class, a nonrequirement, I became familiar with farm crops and could recognize poisonous plants. With a female classmate, I cajoled the university into offering a Reserve Officer Training Corps class on rifles for women. We wanted to learn how to shoot. This was before the days of injectable euthanasia solutions, and large animals that were too sick to recover or had been severely injured by a car were humanely killed with a gun.

I'm concerned that veterinary students today don't have enough close animal contact. A veterinary instructor told me that one good animal case can draw quite a crowd: the instructor, the intern, the resident, the veterinary technician student, and the veterinary technician instructor. "Sometimes I can't get veterinary students close enough to teach them how to duck," he complained. Knowing when to duck is important. If a horse tried to kill me, I wanted to recognize the early warning signals and duck.

In 1959 two women from my class and I applied to veterinary school. Ohio State University had an unofficial quota of three women per class. We heard three women had been accepted, and I thought we had all made it. Then I found out that one of the three women came from West Virginia, a state without a veterinary college. I was first alternate for the class of 1963.

In tears, I sought my favorite animal-science teacher, a champion of women's causes. "Well," he asked, "what are you going to do?"

"Try again," I said.

Adding a third undergraduate year turned out to be the best thing that happened to me. I took a course in cat anatomy with the nurses and also took courses offered in the first year of veterinary school, such as bacteriology and biochemistry. In just three years I earned enough credits for my B.S. in animal science and, in the process, matured.

In 1960 two other women and I were admitted to the freshman class. We became known as the hard-luck class because seventy-two started and only fifty-eight graduated. In the fall of 1960 the Berlin crisis pulled four men into the reserves; others dropped out for various reasons. Having fought so hard to get into veterinary school, my classmates continued to compete with each other that first quarter. Students even moved pointers on practical exams to confuse a classmate. After a few heated class meetings, we realized we would have to pull together to survive the next four years—and we did.

I built a special closeness with my classmates that strengthened senior year in the clinics when we handled a work load intended for a bigger class. Because we depended heavily on each other, no one left the clinic in the evening until all the work was finished. If we weren't the most brilliant class, we were certainly the most industrious. As I look at my classmates, they have done exceptionally well. Many have advanced degrees and board certification.

In those days women weren't allowed to belong to the veterinary fraternity, in which helpful information circulated. We struggled to find equipment that fit, to decide on comfortable work clothes, and to determine how to act. Some of us thought our solutions would help incoming freshmen women. I was one of several women from each class who started *The Link,* a mimeographed newsletter. Its information became a symbolic bridge over the actual river that separated the underclass campus from the veterinary clinics. Students of both sexes from all four years read *The Link.*

I intended to marry a college graduate, but I had no desire to marry a veterinarian. My roommate dated dental students and was always eager to find dates for me. George Clark was one of the blind dates she arranged for me. He graduated from dental school at Ohio State University in June of 1962, and we were married that Christmas, when I was a junior. After his graduation, George reported for active duty in the navy and started a dental internship at Chelsea Naval Hospital in Boston. After a year in Boston, he was assigned to the Everglades, a destroyer tender in Charleston, South Carolina. I stacked up air miles between Boston and Columbus, and Charleston and Columbus.

At first it was a joke, married but living in separate states. At the start of my senior year, I traveled to South Carolina. With my husband assigned to a ship, my first job would have to be in Charleston. Dredging veterinary names from the phone book, I wrote a letter to everyone in town. I told them I would return at Christmas for an interview. Only one veterinarian, Dr. Ernest Horres, responded. He could have paid me anything. I literally begged for the job. I was the first woman veterinarian in Charleston, and I think Ernie's wife accepted me only because I was married.

In Charleston you were considered transient unless your family had been there since the American Revolution. I wasn't just a newcomer—I was *navy*. Ten short days after I arrived, my boss left for a veterinary convention, and I was on my own for forty-five days. Those days still invoke nightmares. Clients flowed through the door all hours of the day and night. We didn't have appointments, and nobody respected business hours. Everyone, it seemed, was related to Ernie or his wife. At six on Saturday night I'd have the key in the lock, and someone with a sick hound would arrive. I'd say, "I'm closed." "But Cousin Ernie always sees me at this time" would be the reply.

As I frantically accumulated experience, I had to face my first loss of a patient and find a way to tell the owner. In school I had performed numerous cesarean sections on cows, but the first one I saw on a dog was the one I was doing. Heartworm disease didn't exist in Ohio, and my school had prepared me neither for the multitude of parasites that thrived in South Carolina nor for the strange fungi that infected animals' skin, ears, and feet. A dog was bitten by a poisonous snake, and frantically I called a neighboring veterinarian for advice. We didn't have poisonous snakes in my part of Ohio. I was so exhausted that if no one talked to me, I'd fall asleep.

I used to drag George along as my anesthetist on late-night emergency calls. Of course, the anesthetic in those days was mostly an ether cone, but George, with his medical background, could evaluate the dog's depth of anesthesia. Once, George helped me wire a fractured mandible on a dog who had been hit by a car. Later George was furious when he learned that the dog's owner gave the dog a bone, and the hearty gnawing broke the wire before the jaw had healed.

Some women had a hard time accepting me as their veterinarian. Dr. Horres spoke soothingly to these women, promising to take care of everything, but I couldn't do that. I decided to talk to them as though we were intelligent women who, together, could solve any problem their pets might develop. I encouraged them to follow my instructions carefully and to keep me informed on the results. If I didn't know a woman's background, I used big words and little words, such as ovariohysterectomy and spay. If I was talking to a head operating-room nurse, I used medical terms. We listened to each other and shared true concern for the pet. Women began to respond, and some even started asking to see me.

During my year in Charleston, an equine encephalitis outbreak took place, and all veterinarians in the area became involved. I was asked to vaccinate some mules on the islands. I could find the people and the mules, but I needed a translator to help me understand Gullah, the difficult island dialect.

In 1965 George was transferred to the Naval Medical Research Institute at the naval medical complex in Bethesda, Maryland, and we moved to Rockville, Maryland. George finished a fellowship and then a master's in biochemistry at George Washington University in Washington, D.C. I found a job with Dr. Alan McEwan in Washington, D.C., in a small-animal practice. I practiced until I was eight months pregnant with my first son, Michael.

In 1968, just before Mike was born, George was assigned to the light cruiser the *Newport News,* whose home port was Norfolk, Virginia. We moved to Virginia Beach, and his ship spent the last part of 1968 and most of 1969 in Vietnam. In Virginia Beach I had a new house with no grass, and as a navy wife I carried the rank and responsibility of my husband. Young officers on George's ship had left behind pregnant wives, and I became a cross between a den mother and a midwife. I took four women to the hospital to have babies and brought them home. I was so busy being mother and navy wife that I didn't miss practice. Nineteen months after I had Michael, Kevin was born.

Two months later, George was reassigned to the Naval Medical Research Institute (NMRI) in Bethesda. He returned to the graduate school at George Washington University to start work on a Ph.D. in biochemistry and do his research at NMRI. We had kept the house in Rockville and simply moved back, this time with two children.

I could train a dog, but I didn't know much about children. Hoping to learn, I participated in a co-op nursery at church. The first day, there were three adults in charge of 20 three-year-olds: the teacher, me, and a man who came in place of his wife, who was having a baby. Soon I discovered that the man was a veterinarian with the federal government. Two parents, two veterinarians. It could probably never happen again.

I had never been a person who liked babies. I wasn't even sure I would like mine, but they were so brilliant, handsome, and clever, I decided to keep them.

When my boys were still in preschool, I returned full-time

to manage the Washington, D.C., practice for one year while the owner recovered from a coronary. My mother came to stay with the boys, and she and her grandsons became very close. After a long day of work, I threw out all those theories about quality of time spent with your children. I had nothing left. I just slept.

Navy responsibilities and work on his Ph.D. kept George so busy that I functioned as a single parent. I don't recall any master plan for raising our boys, but we did try to ingrain two lessons: that it wasn't necessary to be perfect, and that the boys should become self-reliant. As they became older, I tried to show them it was all right to make mistakes by sharing mine with them—even the time I was ripped off by a car dealer. I don't know how to teach self-reliance. Maybe it's like learning to drive. I started the kids in a parking lot and gradually worked up to the expressway. I let them take sheltered risks while I was there to save them. My boys drove in all kinds of weather, even snow so I could monitor their first skid. As young college men, my boys could go around the world on short notice and not blink twice. I wanted self-reliant sons, but sometimes I wish they'd let me do more for them.

When Kevin, the younger son, started kindergarten, I decided to return to work. I'd been out of practice a few years, and changes in drugs and anesthetics placed me in a strange, new world. I was nervous about returning to practice and thought about an alternative career that allowed a regular eight-to-five schedule. My allergist wanted me to stay away from animals. During my second pregnancy my allergies to everything, including animals, became so severe that I was living on corticosteroids. Finally, I accepted a job with the Division of New Drugs in the Food and Drug Administration's Bureau of Veterinary Medicine in Rockville, Maryland.

That ended my practice years. I had expected to like working with animals, but I was surprised at how much I had enjoyed the owners, especially new owners and new puppies. That last year of practice, I remember a client who stuck his head in the exam room door and shouted, "Is that our Dr. Clark, come back?" It felt wonderful to be welcome.

From the standpoint of my career, I can never make up the time lost to shifting jobs and raising children. Male classmates moved ahead of me in money and status.

In 1976 George was assigned to the Naval Dental Research Institute at the Great Lakes Naval Training Center north of Chicago, and I was back in the job market. We moved to Libertyville,

Illinois, and I thought about a federal position in downtown Chicago. At that time I didn't know what a monster Chicago was. A friend told me about an opening for an assistant editor at the American Veterinary Medical Association (AVMA) in Schaumburg, Illinois.

I started at the association as assistant editor under the editor in chief, Dr. Arthur Freeman, in what I thought would be a two-year position. Each month two issues of the *Journal of the American Veterinary Medical Association (JAVMA)* and one issue of the *American Journal of Veterinary Research (AJVR)* were published. I began editing scientific papers for both journals and edited the "What's Your Diagnosis" feature in the *JAVMA*. In the first six months, I thought about quitting a hundred times. What kind of experience did I have for this work? I wasn't a writer. I couldn't spell, except for scientific words. However, I was a critical reader, and this ability was what it took to be a good editor. During my time at Food and Drug, I had developed the ability to evaluate the scientific merit of a report. However, I don't think I ever felt comfortable then or now in the role of editor.

Far from creative writing, scientific papers adhere to a form that readers expect: summary, introduction, materials and methods, results, and discussion. Both journals are refereed, which means people with expertise on a subject review each manuscript. I kept long lists of people with expertise on various subjects related to veterinary medicine. If the reviewers disagreed, I found a third reviewer. However, the editors are the final reviewers.

I may have handled 350 manuscripts a year. Editing a manuscript required total concentration. I felt like I put on a manuscript like I put on a wet suit. My strong basic science background helped me determine if the information made sense. My six years in practice helped me decide if the substance was useful for the majority of readers. Common sense said if an experiment started with fourteen pigs, it should end with fourteen pigs; I didn't care if a pig died or escaped, as long as the author explained what happened. If "this" started a sentence, what "this" referred to had to be clear. An effective editor is a nitpicker with a good memory.

Findings in a scientific report are rarely earth-shattering. Most discoveries are only slight improvements over an existing method. Each report is one small piece in an infinite puzzle.

Editors try to publish articles that are clear, concise, and accurate and won't embarrass the author. Still, printed mistakes are bound in libraries throughout the world and may outlast their authors.

The journals of the AVMA are the two most quoted journals in veterinary medicine. The entire biomedical community references articles from our journals. For veterinarians who must publish to get tenure or sit for specialty boards, our journals are necessary. I'm always pleased when I see young authors grow into tenured faculty.

I try to maintain personal contact with as many people as possible. When an editor from *Cosmopolitan* calls and wants to write an article about women veterinarians under thirty-five years of age in diverse career areas, I can suggest names.

There are about fifty thousand veterinarians in the United States, only enough to fill half of the Ohio State University football stadium. More than 90 percent of these veterinarians belong to the AVMA. As a small association, our members should stay in contact with each other. I think all members should feel they know somebody on our staff in Schaumburg. I always hand out my business card. Although I may have to transfer the call, the member feels that he or she has special clout on headquarters staff. I met a veterinarian at Cornell who mentioned two former instructors I knew. In five minutes we were friends. I have friends all over the country that I have never met.

For the last fifteen years, the AVMA has been evaluating manpower issues. I was involved in initiating a series of journal articles titled "Career Pathways." I recruited authors whose enthusiasm for positions other than private clinical practice bubbled off the page. Trained to be scientists first, veterinarians have a large selection of job possibilities.

In 1981 I was appointed staff adviser to the committee on the human-animal bond. This committee is appointed by the AVMA executive board and represents practicing veterinarians, the university, the government, and the military. I asked to attend the first national meeting on pet loss and euthanasia. The committee developed a client information brochure called "Pet Loss and Human Emotion." They believed that veterinarians could give this brochure to clients struggling with the emotional decision of when to end their pet's life. The brochure was the product of several drafts and the opinions of thirty to forty veterinarians and social scientists. I am very proud that this brochure has turned out to be one of AVMA's best-sellers.

Grieving is a normal expression of loss, whether the loss is a pet or a parent, and local and state veterinary associations sponsor pet-loss support groups. People grieving for their pets are brought together with a clinical psychologist to share their feelings.

The bond between people and animals is enduring. We still discover new ways in which animals add to the quality of human existence. Veterinarians have initiated animal therapy programs in nursing homes, hospitals, and prisons. Horseback riding, for example, can be wonderful therapy for the mentally or physically handicapped. In one nursing home where no pets were allowed, the Boy Scouts built a bird feeder outside a large bay window. Songbirds dined and chirped, to the residents' delight. Even without their own pets, people can feel close to animals. When people see wild geese fly overhead they feel a special kinship. Look at the people touched by the plight of the sea otters in the Alaskan oil spill or by the whales trapped in the arctic ice. During these crises, veterinarians called our office continually to offer their help; the AVMA directed traffic.

In 1989 I made my fourth career change. Now I am the director of AVMA's Career Development Center. The center is in the division of Membership and Field Services and will provide three new member services: computer placement, employment counseling, and opportunities for career expansion in veterinary medicine. These services are geared toward veterinary students, new graduates, veterinarians who have been out of school several years, those looking for mid-career shifts, and others who want to work at something from which they can wind down.

The placement service was activated first. We took this service to several regional veterinary meetings and enlarged our computer files of applicants and employers. At some of these meetings the placement service also arranged personal interviews for interested parties. AVMA members, veterinary students, veterinary technicians, and employers of all types are eligible to use our placement service. A computerized match of applicant and position can be done in three to five working days. Employers receive brief résumés on all appropriate candidates, and applicants are sent a brief description of positions that match their desires and qualifications.

Our counseling service will help veterinarians determine their needs and write accurate résumés. We'll expand career opportunities by becoming the central information source for positions in postgraduate training in basic sciences such as pathology and bacteriology, postdoctoral positions and programs, positions in veterinary schools and science departments, and government preceptorships such as those at the Centers for Disease Control in Atlanta and the National Animal Disease Center in Ames, Iowa.

To attract bright young men and women to our profession, our center will recruit high school students by putting on career days. When the world wakes up to what veterinarians can do, schools won't be able to keep up with the demand.

We are just beginning to realize the importance of our profession. Veterinarians with their broad, multispecies base are fantastic scientists. They escape the narrow human concentration of the physician. Recently the AVMA sponsored a colloquium on diarrheal disease of the young. Physicians as well as veterinarians were present in the audience, and many physicians were speakers. These diseases, often caused by intestinal viruses, threaten not only young animals but also children in impoverished, third world countries. In the United States we can place a sick child in an intensive care unit. This modern technology cannot reach to the middle of the Sahara, where thousands of starving children have diarrheal disease. For years veterinarians have been masters of herd health, controlling disease among a multitude of range cattle, feeder cattle, and swine in confinement housing. They put drugs in the feed and drugs in the water. Veterinarians understand how to treat large groups economically. This is just what people need in developing countries.

I can't believe I now get paid to promote veterinarians. I talk about our diversity. I tell people that our problem-solving skills are our greatest asset. In a pasture, on the range, in the middle of nowhere, there are no supply stores. Even if there were, equipment does not exist that suits all the sizes and shapes and needs of our patients. I remember trying to put a splint on a pony with a fractured hind leg when I was a student. My partner and I held a thick aluminum rod that we intended to bend into a Thomas splint. The first step was to make a circle large enough to encompass the pony's hip. We looked about for a form and spied a telephone pole that was the perfect shape and size. We twisted the rod into a fine-fitting circle. There it remained, irremovable, as testimony to two tired shortsighted students.

Do I ever relax? Not much. I'm a workaholic. If I didn't have to work, I'd work. Long weekends drive me crazy. When George and I were divorced in 1982, I took flying lessons. I needed a diversion and an achievement. A man might buy a car; I earned a pilot's license.

I love to travel. I like to see everything, even Iowa cornfields. Sometimes I combine business with a short vacation. My younger son, Kevin, and I have managed to take a few trips together. Kevin joined me at a meeting in New Orleans, and we explored Bourbon Street together. After a meeting in Boston, Kevin and I drove to Acadia National Park in Maine. My older son, Mike, is in college. He likes to travel on his own, but I get his bills. If someone gave me a long vacation, I'd head for San Francisco, rent a car, and drive up the entire west coast.

I don't know where this job will lead. My mind is on fast-forward. I'm trying not to shoot off in too many directions and get lost. I try to have one continuous list that keeps me organized. I put things on my list to get them out of my head. Veterinarians are interesting people, and I will never tire of being driven by their ideas. ■

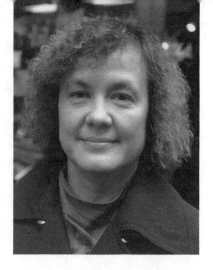

W. Jean Dodds

A CONVERSATION with W. Jean Dodds quickly dispels any notion that research scientists are dull people. As Chief of the Laboratory of Hematology for New York State's Department of Health in Albany, Dodds has conducted and administered comparative research in blood disease for twenty-five years. Known nationally and internationally as an authority on hemostasis, Dodds maintains the largest colony of hemophilic dogs in the world. Testing new drugs first on her dogs, Dodds has provided human hemophiliacs with several breakthrough treatments. Veterinarians recognize her as an expert on all blood diseases, from acquired autoimmune disease to inherited bleeding disorders like von Willebrand's disease.

As a comparative hematologist, Dodds commands equal authority in human medicine. She has earned the political clout to joust with others in the medical hierarchy on numerous policymaking committees, in which she represents the veterinary viewpoint for the welfare of all research animals.

"It should be the goal of everybody in biomedical teaching not to have to use animals for research," she says. "This cannot occur in the foreseeable future,

because whole animals are necessary to complete observations begun with nonanimal techniques. Presently, in the pool of research money, animals have too low a priority. I argue for a higher priority for animals. Federal regulations already require scientists to consider alternative techniques. I emphasize this point by appealing to human conscience to save life and, by so doing, actually save money. Alternative techniques cost less than using live animals."

Graduating with honors and distinction in 1964 from the Ontario Veterinary College at the University of Guelph, Dodds continued the research program she had been involved in as a student by accepting the position of research scientist for the New York State Department of Health. In 1983 she advanced to become the director of hematology for the department and supervised the state's human blood banks.

Dodds has been honored with the following awards: Woman Veterinarian of the Year (1974), awards for outstanding service to the veterinary profession from the American Animal Hospital Association (1977–1978), Gaines Fido Award, as dogdom's Woman of the Year (1978), Centennial Medal Award, University of Pennsylvania, School of Veterinary Medicine (1984). In 1987 she was elected Distinguished Practitioner of the National Academy of Practice in Veterinary Medicine. Moving to California in 1986 to capitalize on that state's propensity for invention, Dodds relinquished her New York success to concentrate on her professional goal, a national blood bank for animals.

"My father was a brilliant medical doctor but nevertheless a cynic who instilled in me the philosophy that to be accepted, I had to excel," Dodds says. "At the top, he told me, I would have power over everyone else because I'd proved I was better. All my life I struggled with his belief. I wondered, Why can't a person do well because she cares to do well and is not putting anybody down, just doing her own thing, finding her own space? So I tried very hard to understand why people do the things they do. Even if I disagreed with them, I tried to be more tolerant. I didn't change my basic value system, but by understanding the opposition, I became a better adversary. Feeling that my values represented care, compassion, and love gave me the fortitude to use all means necessary, as long as they didn't hurt others, to make myself effective."

■

Anything I've really wanted to do in life that's meaningful hasn't come easy. I've had to stand up and fight for it.

I was born in Shanghai, China. My mother's family were British merchants in Shanghai, and my father's parents were missionaries with the Plymouth Brethren. I was about six months old when my parents escaped on the last boat to leave Shanghai before the Japanese internment in 1941.

Descended from a long line of medical people, Father earned his medical degree in Canada. While he was finishing his internship and residency in Toronto, I was just old enough to have snowball fights with my sister, one and a half years younger. When Father's schooling was completed, he took an assignment in Hong Kong to work for the World Health Organization. My sister and I grew up in the Hong Kong school system. When we reached our first year of high school, Father decided his children should have some feeling for their native country, so we returned to Canada. While I was in high school, Father traveled to Maryland to finish his doctorate in public health at Johns Hopkins University. Afterwards he became director of Indian and Eskimo affairs for the Canadian government. We lived in Montreal two years, then in Ottawa.

In the early 1950s, Canada was not as socially aware as the United States, but coming from Hong Kong, where my sister and I wore starched uniforms to school, we looked very old-fashioned to the Canadians. We were eggheads. We thought studying was what you were supposed to do. We didn't wear makeup, and we didn't date. Of course, we were ostracized. To win acceptance, my sister and I became athletes, good enough in all the sports to play on teams that won regional championships.

I always wanted to be a veterinarian. Even in China our family had many pets—cats and dogs—but my great love was horses. Only the very rich had horses in Hong Kong, and in Canada we were urbanites. I indulged my horse fancies by memorizing all the winners of the Kentucky Derby and later keeping detailed, up-to-date racing records for harness and flat tracks. As a veterinary student, I bet on the horses for recreation. I'd spend three or four dollars and come home with fifty. Once, at a raceway in Yonkers, New York, I missed the fourteen-hundred-dollar payoff by one horse. Coming so close to riches, I could feel the obsession of gambling, so I stopped. I couldn't let money control me.

When we came to Canada from Hong Kong, I was ordinary and shy, with straight fine hair, assertive in a quiet sort of way because I wasn't as confident then as I am now. There wasn't much to like about myself, and I wished I wasn't so driven to succeed. At home Father's love seemed to flow in proportion to his children's excellence.

My father was an unusual person, enormously intelligent and successful but very hard to be with. He was the ultimate chauvinist; women didn't count. In his eyes, daughters were acceptable as long as they excelled academically, and he rewarded us with money—not much, but the intent was clear. My brother, seven years younger, was the son from which Father's medical genes would succeed. Father heaped a great deal of hope and aspiration on my brother, who finally rebelled and dropped out of medical school after two years. Yet if Father hadn't instilled in all his children this sense of purpose, of working very hard to achieve, then none of us would probably have been as successful as we were. My sister became deputy minister of customs and excise for the Canadian government, and my brother now owns his own printing and publishing company outside Toronto.

For a while Father encouraged me to be a veterinarian. Then he insisted I become a physician. If I liked animals because they didn't talk, I should be a pediatrician. He did not want his oldest daughter associated with an uncouth profession that dealt with beasts and feces; certainly that was pseudomedicine with pseudoscientists. According to my father's ill-founded stereotype, farmers couldn't be intellectuals, because they worked with their hands. He felt such people would waste my intelligence. When I persisted, he finally blamed a woman relative, a naturalist who painted watercolors of animals, for tainting his medical genes.

One Easter holiday, in the pouring rain, Father drove me to Guelph to tour the Ontario Veterinary College. He assured me that I would see for myself that veterinary medicine was not for me. At that time Guelph had the most progressive large-animal surgery arena in North America. Through expansive glass windows we watched operating tables tilt and the floor rise to allow a powerful horse to be securely fastened to the table. Surgeons scrubbed and wore gowns, caps, and masks just like their medical counterparts. Father was astounded, and my eyes grew huge. Before we left, I enrolled in the class of 1964. The competition to enter was stiff, and I didn't expect to be accepted, but just in case, I gave them my name and résumé.

"Damn it!" Father said on the drive home. "I brought you to prove that veterinary medicine wasn't for you, and now I've convinced you more than ever to be a veterinarian. Well, perhaps you'd better be one."

Mother had a basic university degree and was administrator of the biology department at York University. Unlike Father, she was fond of animals. She always believed her children should do their own thing.

Entrance requirements at Guelph were farm experience and high grades. Whatever they wanted, I did. I had to be a veterinarian. For two summers I lived on farms, stooked grain, and milked cows. The veterinary college had a quota of twenty women total, for all five years. If two graduated, they accepted two freshmen. Despite these restrictions, I now felt very sure about being accepted.

In 1959 I became one of four freshman women in the Ontario Veterinary College. One of these young women became pregnant and, according to university rules, had to leave. Another decided to become a physician, so two new women joined us at the end of freshman year.

When I came home the summer after we studied anatomy, Father was incredulous. "You can't possibly know the anatomy of all those species to the extent that we do in medical school," he said.

"It's too much to learn."

"We do too," I said.

He pointed to his leg. "What's this muscle? What's the nerve? What's the vessel?"

I rattled off the names.

He stared at me. "I'm very impressed."

Father brought home anesthetic and asked me to remove a plantar wart on his foot. Mother tried to intervene. "I'll remove it," she said.

"No. Jean will," Father insisted.

After I finished cutting out his wart, Father wrote me a little receipt: paid in full for service, one dollar.

My first student controversy involved large-animal clinics. We had three Nigerians in our class, royalty from some reciprocal program. They were small men, very black with piercing white eyes, impressively clever, and very polite, but terrified of large animals. The college considered waiving their clinic requirement, but if these "delicate men" were excused, what about the women? The college decided that we were all to graduate as equals, so we would all participate in clinics. I remember a practical exam in clinic that required each student to put a mouth gag in a heifer. After the poor beast had been wrestled by thirty students, it was my turn. When I grabbed the heifer, she began to fight for her freedom. I don't remember ever being so physically exhausted, but I got the gag in. The other women were less successful, and the Nigerians would not even try.

In surgery, women were made to wear white pants and the same see-through T-shirts the men wore. Our bras showed, and the men enjoyed class too much. We held a women's meeting and decided to buy our own nurse uniforms. When they arrived, the dean refused permission to wear them. I wore mine anyway. The first day in my new white dress, I raced along the slippery marble hall, trying not to be late. Swinging around a corner, I smacked into a professor's stomach.

"Good God, woman," he said, "what are you doing in your slip?"

"Sir! My slip? This is my new nurse's outfit."

"Oh, very nice," he said.

The physiology laboratory was old and had a wooden stage where the same professor stood to draw diagrams on a blackboard. The girls were made to sit in the front row. One day the old exposed pipes in the ceiling burst and sprayed hot rusty water on us. The women had been so humiliated and dominated that they wouldn't squeak, let alone do anything to draw attention to themselves. So I flopped on the stage in front of the professor.

"What are you doing?" he shouted.

"Look! There's hot rusty water falling on us!"

"My God! Why don't the rest of you girls move?"

My clinic partner was a small fellow from Nova Scotia, who tended to strut, trying to be tall. He made it known that his only interest was large-animal medicine because small-animal doctors were regarded as sissies. In the small-animal clinics, I spent a lot of time talking to animals, gentling them and taking dogs for walks so they would feel better and recover faster. I explained this theory to my partner. When he thought no one was looking, he also played with the dogs and cats. His classmates noticed but dared not talk about it. At graduation my partner received the small-animal clinic award for the student with the most compassion. He blamed me and is probably still annoyed.

At graduation three women, myself included, ranked among the top ten students. The head of ambulatory service, a man I greatly admired, looked at the three of us during his graduation speech and made it very clear he felt women had no place in large-animal medicine.

I loved animals and wanted to care for them, but I always saw myself in research. A general practice seemed too limited. In research, I could aim toward important discoveries that I hoped would translate to a practice setting and be used to save lives. Father liked my decision. He saw research as comparative medicine in which I dealt with humankind as well as animals. His daughter had rejoined the intellectuals.

In college I supported myself with the help of a scholarship and stayed on campus in summer to job-hunt. The pathophysiology laboratory advertised for help but wouldn't hire a woman because, as the professor in charge told me, the last female student they'd hired dressed like a man and slept in the ladies' washroom with her German shepherd. The head of the pathophysiology division had been my father's classmate at Johns Hopkins University. I mentioned my father's name to see if I could gain an advantage. In the midst of recalling old memories, H. C. Rowsell hired me to work at the research station down the road from the veterinary school. My hemostasis work with a colony of dogs began that summer of 1960, at the end of my freshman year. Dr. Rowsell was my role model and became my close friend and colleague. When I attended class, I ran the research project part-time. The year I graduated, 1964, I became assistant professor of physiology at Ontario Veterinary College.

The dog colony had been funded by the U.S. National Institutes of Health (NIH), which in 1965 withdrew eligibility for routine application to foreign countries like Canada. The New York State Department of Health invited us to transfer our project and bring our dog colony to Albany to continue work on hemostasis and atherosclerosis. We had a newly funded NIH grant totaling one million dollars. I was offered a position as research scientist for the Department of Health, and the two senior research doctors were offered positions across the street at Albany Medical College. Everyone, I thought, had decided to go. I transported the most valuable dogs and two laboratory technicians to New York and rented a house adjacent to the department's research farm. There I organized a research laboratory from nothing, not even a test tube. At the last minute the two senior investigators decided to stay in Canada. I was abandoned with a dog colony and a $7,800-a-year job with the health department.

I was a kid, out of school one year. I immediately petitioned NIH to continue that portion of the funds for what was now my dog colony. The physicians I'd worked with wrote NIH in my behalf and said I'd done all the work with the dogs. I still remember the feeling when NIH called. "We're sorry we can't fund your program for seven years," the official said, "but we'll give you all the money you need for two years. After that you have to reapply."

I was elated. They only wanted me to prove myself. We could do that. We'd been doing that. I grabbed their challenge and built the dog colony into a multimillion-dollar program that's still operating with me as the principal investigator.

Hemostasis research was just starting in the 1960s, and over the years it developed from a general field into highly sophisticated molecular biology in which blood proteins are cloned artificially. It is very rare when a field in science and medicine like hematology undergoes so many complex changes during one professional lifetime. In the beginning, when little was known, I learned by trial and error, a very tedious, very difficult, very challenging method. By choosing this undeveloped discipline, I became an expert by exclusion. I've accumulated and contributed to knowledge that has saved many human and animal lives.

Our dog colony, now the largest colony of hemophiliacs in the world, has always been the heart of my research. Dogs are the only animal species affected with the same range of inherited bleeding diseases as humans. Everything we learn about detection, treatment, and control can be applied directly to human medicine.

We keep between 80 and 120 dogs of all breeds in special runs designed to prevent trauma. The worst bleeders live in pens on deep piles of cedar wood shavings. The dogs aren't permitted to roughhouse with each other, and we monitor them closely for signs of bleeding. Owners often give us their dogs because they know we allow them to live relatively normal lives with a disease that is potentially fatal. With all we've learned about hemophilia, it still cannot be cured. It makes me humble to realize that a dog that appears healthy one minute can be dead from hemorrhage in a few hours.

Although many purebred dogs carry genes for hemophilia (the females) or other bleeding diseases (either sex), the actual disease is expressed in a relatively small percentage of the general dog population. Von Willebrand's disease, however, is much more common in both dogs and people than true hemophilia and can be either inherited or acquired. A clot is slow to form, and the bleeding tendency becomes especially critical during surgery and other periods of stress. In my early research, I discovered that my mother and I had a mild form of von Willebrand's disease. We've always bruised easily. Mother almost bled to death when she gave birth to my sister. I hemorrhaged severely from a tonsillectomy. The von Willebrand factor is a plasma protein that makes the surface of blood platelets sticky so they initiate hemostasis. Excessive bleeding occurs when this factor is missing.

My work with the dog colony allows me to collaborate with scientists in molecular biology who have recently cloned some of the plasma proteins responsible for blood coagulation. Once the artificially produced proteins were proven safe in small laboratory animals, we injected some of these products into our dogs. The dogs responded well, with no side effects, so the new clotting factors now are being used in clinical trials in humans. When this method is perfected, hemophiliacs won't have to rely on transfusions from blood donors and take that small inherent risk of disease. Yet whole plasma will never be replaced in the clinic because it contains other important proteins, like albumen and globulins, that can't be efficiently produced by artificial means. As we learn more about hemostasis, we also solve the opposite mystery: blood that coagulates too rapidly and thromboses or blocks small blood vessels.

Some of our research is labeled controversial, and skeptical scientists are surprised when we eventually produce expected results. High-quality research is not voodoo. Our team abides by conventional rules: voracious reading, detailed preparation, persistence, and creativity. Our search for answers creates new knowledge.

I've been called a scientific psychic. We accept referral cases on a national basis, so my associates and I see more abnormal hematology cases—one hundred in a year—than a practitioner who sees one case or a veterinary college clinician who sees five cases. Our large caseload makes certain trends evident. I have called the Animal Medical Center in New York and asked, "Aren't you seeing more kidney and liver disease in these last five years than in the previous ten?" They look and also see the trend, which cannot be ascribed to increased awareness or better diagnostic tests. Now we're all scientific psychics.

Our research on autoimmune disease focuses on four major causes: genetic predisposition, hormones (especially thyroid), infections (especially viral), and stress. When we examine animals, we consider all tissues—blood and bone marrow, the liver, the kidney, et cetera. A change in any body organ will eventually affect the blood. Hematology and immunology are closely related; viral exposure or infection changes the white blood cells that protect against disease. Hypothyroidism causes changes in the immune system associated with bleeding. My own referral cases with acquired immune-mediated hemolytic anemia or thrombocytopenia often respond to thyroid medication and proper diets. Autoimmune thyroiditis can lead to problems with other tissues, including the blood and bone marrow, so we minimize use of steroids after the initial phase of the disease is controlled.

Preventive medicine is the key to disease control. Veterinarians need to become so familiar with normal patterns of blood proteins, chemistry, and cellular components that they can very early detect imbalances likely to progress to organ failure. Pet owners must be taught to request annual physical examinations with proper laboratory tests, and they must provide thorough medical and family histories. This is critical to early interception of disease. Presently a veterinarian sees many cases in an advanced stage when less can be done.

Some veterinarians don't believe people will pay a hundred dollars or more for a yearly health screen on their pets. I ask dog breeders, "You'll pay to keep your dogs healthy, won't you?" Sure, veterinarians double the price of a laboratory test, but that extra money pays for technician overhead, the cost of the hospital, and the doctor's time. The doctor must at least break even to provide the service. Pet owners who understand the cost system and believe that their pet needs a health profile will pay for it. If I can persuade small groups of dog breeders to request this more sophisticated service, veterinarians will gladly fill the demand. Eventually the health profile will spill over into other animal groups.

I ask veterinarians, "How would you like to have intravenous gamma globulins available, sterile, and ready to use at a reasonable cost, to treat puppies dying from parvovirus disease or calves infected with colibacillosis?"

"Sounds great! Where can I get some?" is the reply.

There's an incredible need for blood and plasma derivatives in clinical veterinary medicine. Medical doctors use them to strengthen the human immune system or replace missing components, but veterinarians don't yet realize the value of plasma proteins, white cells, and platelets. These elements have never been available. They could be available if the veterinarian and the consumer demand them. When requests pour in, some drug company will see a product that can be profitable.

In the next decade, pet insurance will become more important. The average pet owner cannot pay two thousand dollars or more for total hip replacement. If the cost of veterinary services runs between two hundred and one thousand dollars, a large number of people cannot afford them and may choose to euthanize their pet. We need insurance to cover catastrophic illness and chronic disease whose treatment can cost into the thousands.

Cancer therapy alone can cost a fortune. Veterinary medicine uses sophisticated CAT scans, radiation therapy, and complicated chemotherapy protocols. Oncologic treatment is an ethical dilemma for me because it often buys only three or four months of time for the animal. Life is prolonged beyond what I think is in the animal's best interest; it's mostly the owner's needs that are being appeased. I saw a cat with nasal carcinoma, for example. The tumor had been irradiated, and half of the cat's face was missing; only the bones remained. It was pathetic. I believe we have to look at the quality and dignity of a pet's life and reach a point where we refuse to continue treatment. Reasonable owners choose euthanasia when they realize their pet is suffering with no hope of recovery.

With my busy career, my personal life at times has been hectic. In my second year of veterinary school I married Jim Dodds, a veterinary student one class ahead of me, and divorced him the day I graduated. Having a child was unthinkable because pregnant students were asked to drop out.

After five years of freedom, I married my immunology professor at Albany Medical College. He was older than I, was supporting an ex-wife and four children, and certainly had no need for more children. He was very successful at Albany, was respected for his ideas and acknowledged for his abilities, and had been awarded Teacher of the Year. We were married in 1969 when I was a new discovery in hematology and public health. Wherever hematology was debated, I was invited as one of the scientific experts. I traveled all over the world, and my husband accompanied me as "Mr. Dodds." The vitality of my growing career overpowered my husband's success and began to destroy his sense of self-worth. At home I found time to paint, wallpaper, and tackle simple household repairs. I wanted to be the perfect cook, the perfect housewife. Even these simple activities annoyed my husband. Our areas of mutual pleasure and agreement shrank until we were incompatible. Finally we divorced.

My first two marriages were mistakes. I chose men who resembled my father and wanted to dominate me. I believe I wanted another chance to earn my father's love. I tried to change myself but I couldn't.

After remaining single for twelve years, I married a man who knew me well and loved me. Charles Berman is a patent attorney, accomplished and self-assured. He met me when I gave expert testimony for Cedar Sinai Hospital. We are both Orthodox Jews and were married in 1986 in an Orthodox ceremony. We communicate totally, and this makes my personal life extremely happy.

My family was always religiously unsettled. Father's parents were zealots in the strict Quaker sense, so, in rebellion, my father declared himself an atheist. My search for religious stability led me to study Orthodox Judaism. After one and a half years of study, I felt that I could accept these beliefs and that they would help me function more effectively. I converted to Orthodox Judaism. In his retirement, my father writes about ancient religions based on original Hebrew scripture. By chance we both study Judaism.

Charles and I are both vegetarians. Judaism and our diet exist nicely together. We don't have to worry about separating meat and milk in our kitchen. I stopped eating veal first, because of my concern for the kind of life calves live before they are killed. Factory farming—raising animals indoors in close confinement—does not allow an animal to lead a normal life. It is cost-effective, but I don't believe money should be the driving force of agriculture. If we choose to eat animals, our prime responsibility is to allow that animal to enjoy life. We must give livestock freedom to move inside and outside and provide humane shipping conditions before humane slaughter. After slaughter, we should use the whole carcass, even process the hide for leather.

After veal, I gave up red meat. I had enjoyed an occasional steak, but my favorite meat was chicken and turkey (kosher, of course). Once a month when I was in Albany to supervise our research program, I would stay at a local rabbi's home. His wife served delicious, crunchy, fried kosher chicken. I enjoyed her chicken long after I'd given up poultry at home and in kosher restaurants. To be less of a hypocrite, I now eat only kosher fish (no shellfish) and animal by-products like eggs, milk, and kosher cheese. I've been a vegetarian five years and now find even the smell of meat repulsive. In restaurants I usually ask for a plate of vegetables, and if I crave variety, I find that salad, bread, potatoes, rice, and pasta are always plentiful. On New Year's Day I served poached salmon and fettuccine Alfredo. As vegetarians, Charles and I believe we have improved our health and vigor. Even if the farmer improves animal care, I would not change. I cannot sacrifice a life for my sustenance when healthy alternatives are available.

Once I spent a whole day at San Diego Zoo, where animals live in an ideal environment. After several hours I became melancholy because I saw no spark in the animals' eyes. They reminded me of the hundreds of people who quickly ebb and flow when the bullet train stops in Tokyo. These people look so uniform and robotlike. Highly regimented populations all have the same apathy in their eyes. If people are pushed too fast, controlled too much, are they really free? Maybe zoo animals would prefer the uncertain life of the wild.

Wild animals are very important, because I'm convinced humans are dependent on the world's ecology. As we become more withdrawn and isolated from nature, we take away the evolutionary concept of our being. Judaism gives humankind dominion over animals, but we must make decisions with compassion, using our intelligence and talents to relieve pain and suffering.

All living animals have equal value. I could, however, more easily take the life of a mouse than that of a dog or cat. It's not rational, just personal preference.

I still travel a great deal, talking to groups who are interested in improving animal welfare. Taxpayer dollars are spent to develop my career, so I feel people deserve some return. I speak to fanciers of purebred dogs and find these people receptive to new ideas. Healthy show dogs make their owners a success, so these people try to amass considerable information about their breed. Most purebreds have been linebred and inbred so much that all are genetically similar. Without starting over, all I can do to control serious inherited problems is to teach breeders to eliminate factors that cause expression of genetic predisposition, like how to breed out familial autoimmune thyroid disease and provide proper nutrition, health, and lower stress. Some breeders intimidate veterinarians when they challenge the veterinarians' knowledge. To work with breeders' dogs, veterinarians must get through this personality barrier. Once hooked, breeders make very faithful clients. I breed vizslas and pointers, do a little match or specialty judging, and have many breeder friends and clients.

The ability to communicate with animals is innate, but it can be somewhat learned. I try to explain to my husband, who's had very little animal contact, that animals are more intelligent than most people realize. Our body language and words communicate our feelings to animals, and if a person is tuned in, animals in turn tell us what they need. Once a person understands animals, they discover that no two dogs are alike. I approach my patients gently, talk to them, and touch them in a way that implies trust. If people show fear, they discourage an animal's friendship. I recall receiving only one dog bite, from a Chihuahua who didn't want his nails trimmed.

My mother and I moved to Santa Monica, California, in 1986 when I married Charles. I still consult on difficult blood cases from all over the country. California state laws say I must have a license to practice as a consultant because I reside there. This means that I would have to pass both the national board examination and the California state exam—twenty-six years after graduation. Up to a year's time would be spent updating myself in large-animal and other medicine. Most of this knowledge I would never use, so I feel it would be time wasted. I could much more easily pass an examination about general small-animal or laboratory medicine. I am a good example of the need for limited licenses, a license restricted to a specialty like hematology, ophthalmology, internal medicine, or an animal group, like large-animal, small-animal, or exotics. To change specialties, a veterinarian would get a limited license by passing a competency test on necessary information.

Currently, our veterinary licensure system has no such options. Medical doctors are licensed for certain specialties, and it's time for the veterinary profession to update its thinking. At least the American Veterinary Medical Association is discussing the issue. Fifteen years ago it wouldn't even put limited licensure on the agenda.

As a research veterinarian involved equally in human and animal medicine, I'm very concerned about the use of animals in biomedical research. It seems I've been on every national committee dealing with this subject. I was appointed by the National Academy of Sciences under a congressional mandate to represent veterinary medicine, laboratory-animal medicine, and comparative research by serving on a committee with the world's most prestigious physicians. At this level, men have rarely encountered a qualified woman and had to seriously consider her opinion. I was one of two women, and some of these men stereotyped us as having less backbone and too much emotion to regard animal issues on an intellectual, scientific basis.

High-level medical administrators are usually anti-regulation because universities and medical institutions are regulated to death. Each new regulation adds paperwork, people, computer time, and more cost. Scientists find it hard to concentrate on their goal, which is to complete meaningful research to advance knowledge. Instead they are tied up by regulations only peripherally related to their research.

The animal welfare regulations currently in effect are adequate to protect research animals when enforced not to the letter but to the underlying principle. People cannot be regulated 100 percent, but they can be encouraged to think.

I promote use of alternative techniques to live animals. When animals aren't used, money is saved. My views for reasonable protection of laboratory animals usually side with the minority. To be included and allowed to express my opinion where it counts, I have learned to overlook bruises to my ego and to retreat to a middle ground. Here I can remain effective, and if my views are not totally accepted, at least I can neutralize some of medicine's more dogmatic fears.

With my success in public health, administration duties claimed a greater portion of my time. I could no longer remain competent in both public health and veterinary research. Time for my dog colony was crowded out. I always wanted to work with people through animals, but I seemed to be getting farther away from veterinary medicine. I had to ask myself if this was the direction I wanted to go. What was the most important thing in my life?

I made an appointment with New York's commissioner of health, who should be disturbed only for matters of seismic proportion.

"It's time for your fledgling to fly," I told him. "I want to do something different with my life."

He was very calm. "Tell me what you want to do."

"I feel bad about wanting to do something for myself, because I'll be letting people down who have worked with me in this program twenty-five years," I said. "The program is entirely dependent on me for funding."

He slapped his desk with his palm. "Don't ever say you can't make a decision for something you need because other people are depending on you. For years afterward you will blame yourself for letting them force you to do what you didn't want to do. Do what you have to, and after a while others will understand."

"I must return to veterinary medicine," I said, "but I want to continue here half-time, helping and encouraging my staff in their transition period."

"That's fine," he said. "Things will work out."

In California I began my not-for-profit national blood bank for animals. For the first year and a half, I returned to New York every two weeks to personally direct research with my dog colony. Now I visit every four to six weeks. The rest of the time, I supervise by telephone, photocopier, and fax machines.

The people of California are eager to invest in new ideas. They give me breathing room and encouragement to try something that's never been done before. My company, Hemopet, is still an infant. Mother and I distribute blood bags and collection equipment at cost. We will send as little as one blood collection bag to a practitioner or will supply volumes to large veterinary centers like the San Diego Emergency Clinic. Now I send bags containing anticoagulant, but soon I will be able to supply typed whole blood and components. A great need exists, but first I must work out an efficient and safe system to supply the demand without exploiting the donor animals. To satisfy animal activists and my personal concerns proves to be quite an intellectual challenge.

Constantly searching for answers, I have at last created harmony in my spiritual, private, and professional life. I still travel too much, but it's important for me to teach people to improve the care of their animals. I don't charge for my advice, because I so enjoy giving it.

It is clear that animals suffer. Encouraging compassionate care is the veterinarian's first responsibility. ■

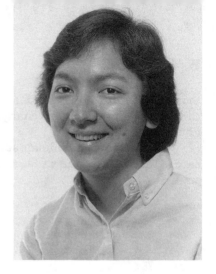

Margaret Gourlay

AT 10 P.M. Margaret Gourlay, a small woman in her mid-twenties, walked quietly through the wards, checking on patients and administering medications at the Iowa State University Veterinary Teaching Hospital in Ames. At the time she was interviewed for this book, Gourlay was a senior veterinary student, and her duties for night emergency call required an overnight stay at the hospital. Between treating and admitting patients, Gourlay discussed her experiences and aspirations.

A woman of many interests and talents, Gourlay loves writing as well as veterinary medicine and had a hard time deciding between the two career directions. She successfully merged the two disciplines by serving as business manager of the *Iowa State University Veterinarian* and as the 1988–1989 editor of *Intervet,* the journal of the Student American Veterinary Medical Association (SAVMA).

Gourlay is also an active participant in SAVMA and other college organizations, as well as the recipient of numerous awards and scholarships, including the Pearl Hogrefe Fellowship Award in Creative Writing. In spite of her accomplishments, Gourlay has an unassuming nature. That and her excellent listening skills will serve her well in veterinary practice, her goal after graduation.

■

My dad is a veterinarian. He graduated from Cornell University in the 1950s and met my mom, who was a secretary, when he was stationed in Korea in the Army. My parents were both in their thirties when they married and were anxious to have a family, I think. My older sister, Linda, was born in Seoul, and one and a half years later, I was born in Bangkok. When I was a year old, our family moved to the United States.

Dad enjoyed regulatory veterinary medicine and hoped to find a civilian regulatory position with the government. Before he returned to the United States, he wrote to Dr. W. A. Hagan, the original director of the National Animal Disease Center (NADC) and the former dean of the Cornell Veterinary College, concerning employment opportunities. Dr. Hagan hired Dad at NADC in Ames, Iowa, and that's where I grew up.

Dad was employed at NADC in vaccine evaluation, and I remember him working with test tubes rather than animals. He was involved in the testing and licensing of the first canine parvovirus vaccines when parvovirus was pandemic in the United States in the late 1970s. After twenty-two years of regulatory work, Dad retired and at the present time serves as a consultant for companies seeking licenses for veterinary vaccines.

My parents are divorced now. My dad has remarried and lives in California, and my mom lives in Minneapolis. My older sister is a nurse practitioner in Iowa City. We like to joke that Mom and Dad flew from the nest and left us kids in Iowa.

89

Because I am half Korean, I look a little different and people are always guessing that I am Chinese, Spanish, or even French. I wish now that my family had blended more of the oriental culture with the American. When my sister and I were young, Mom made a feeble attempt to teach us to write and speak Korean, but we did so poorly that she gave up. Mom stayed at home as a traditional housewife. In the Korean culture, the role of wife and mother is taken very seriously and given more status than in our culture.

I always looked up to my dad. He is one of the most objective people I know. He never pushed my sister or me one way or the other. When I was a little girl, I remember telling him that I wanted to be a fireman, and with a straight face, he said, "Fine." When I said I wanted to be a veterinarian, he reacted in much the same way, but I really think he was excited about it.

I look to Dad for advice. We talk a lot about what I'm going to do after graduation. I've discussed with him my interest in entering the Peace Corps someday. He said that his overseas experience with the Army was wonderful. However, a new graduate will not have his or her veterinary skills challenged as much in an underdeveloped country, and many veterinarians fresh out of school need to solidify those skills. He can troubleshoot with me out of his experience.

I always thought about becoming a veterinarian. However, it became a battle between the sciences and the humanities for me in high school and college. I love English and writing, and it was extremely hard to decide between veterinary medicine and writing. I finally decided that I could be a veterinarian and write on the side, but I couldn't figure out a way to be a full-time author and practice veterinary medicine on the side. Writing skills have a practical value for veterinarians who are writing research reports or designing a clinic newsletter, but the main reason I write is for the sense of enjoyment it brings me.

I started college at Iowa State University to get my preveterinary requirements out of the way. After my sophomore year, I transferred to the University of Iowa in Iowa City. The University of Iowa offers a fantastic graduate writing program, the Iowa Writers' Workshop, which is world-famous.

I took five years to complete my bachelor's degree. I majored in microbiology with an English minor. It was an ideal balance, allowing me to switch back and forth between the sciences and the humanities. One of my honors English classes required us to keep a journal. I loved that journal because it was an outlet for creativity and because it offered a way to escape from the competitive atmosphere of the preveterinary curriculum.

During my last two years at the University of Iowa, I enrolled in fewer classes so I could work to help pay tuition and expenses. I was a research assistant in the Radiation Biology Department and supervised four laboratory assistants. I reported to a postdoctoral fellow who designed the experiments, primarily in the immunology field. It was neat to have a project and not know how it was going to turn out. I liked that element of mystery. Sometimes the project had to be redesigned as we went along. I took blood samples, gave injections, and performed elementary surgery and dissection on rats and mice. When I got to veterinary school, I had a working knowledge of lab animals and research.

Starting in high school and continuing through my sophomore year in college, I was an animal caretaker in the clinics at the veterinary school. I wanted to gain exposure to the clinical side of veterinary medicine. The summer following my first year in veterinary school, I worked for All Pets Veterinary Clinic in Iowa City. I administered medications and fluids, cleaned and sterilized instruments, performed basic lab tests, and bathed and groomed animals.

The following summer, between my second and third years in veterinary school, I worked as a laboratory aide in the brucellosis research unit at the National Animal Disease Center. Also, for three and a half weeks at the beginning of that summer, I participated in an International Veterinary Student Association exchange to Blackburn, England.

Through the exchange program, I worked for three veterinarians who operated a small-animal hospital in Blackburn, a town with a population of 100,000, near the northern border. The practice was housed in an old building and didn't seem as commercialized as some of the practices I had observed in the States. We didn't vaccinate against rabies, because Great Britain is rabies-free. The English veterinarians are called Mister instead of Doctor, and the veterinary technicians are called animal nurses. Several young people—elementary and junior high school age—also rotated through the practice. It was an opportunity for the kids to see the real world of work in their areas of interest. Young people in that country are encouraged at an early age to think about careers.

I had wonderful experiences, and my knowledge was

respected. About a week into the exchange, I followed one of the practitioners into an exam room and was surprised when he announced to the client that I would be giving Fido his vaccination. After two weeks, the practitioner had me scrubbing up and assisting in surgery. I learned something from each of the veterinarians in the practice and had a great time.

While I was in England, I visited the author James Herriot, who is James Alfred Wight in real life. I had written Mr. Herriot ahead of time, and he wrote back and suggested that I call him when I could schedule a visit. I rang his office number and was shocked when he answered the telephone.

James Herriot sees callers at his surgery in Thirby, Thirsk, two afternoons each week. About thirty of us, mostly Americans, went in to see him. The veterinary practice was very unobtrusive, and there was no large sign at the entrance. Townspeople, paying no attention to us visitors, walked into and out of the surgery with their pets while we waited to see Mr. Herriot.

James Herriot is in his seventies and still is practicing and writing. He is the nicest man. You feel like you could sit down and talk to him all day. He is a prolific letter writer, and I will always treasure the letters I received from him.

I have all of his books. He is a skillful author and a real people-watcher. You can tell he loves people, as well as animals. This is an important part of being a veterinarian. You aren't just dealing with an animal—there's a person behind the animal, too.

I don't think the general public was aware of what veterinarians really did until the Herriot books. I've heard that the great increase in numbers of applicants to veterinary schools in the 1970s was due at least in part to his books.

I will graduate from veterinary school in 1990. In my class of 102 students, 43 are women. I have been unaware of any major barriers based on gender, and I've had a lot of male as well as female professors whom I consider role models.

When I was editor of *Intervet,* I wrote an editorial about mentors. To me, the most important quality in a mentor or role model is the ability to give advice while still allowing the other person to learn by making his or her own decisions and mistakes.

The *Iowa State University Veterinarian* is the student publication at our veterinary school. I was in charge of the budget from 1986 to 1987. One of the reasons I took the job was to develop my skills in the area of business and accounting. It was very good training for *Intervet,* the publication for the Student American Veterinary Medical Association (SAVMA). I have been active in SAVMA since I started veterinary school. Representatives of SAVMA meet twice a year, at the American Veterinary Medical Association national convention and at alternating veterinary schools.

Usually, student representatives from the various veterinary schools bid for handling *Intervet.* However, during the 1987 spring symposium at Colorado State University, no one competed for the publication. I came back to Iowa State and talked to students and faculty about bidding for the journal. I thought it was something that we could do for SAVMA. The student body here got very excited about it, and more than one hundred veterinary students volunteered to help. We bid against Ohio State University and obtained the *Intervet* assignment for the 1988–89 school year.

I thought that I could make time to be the editor because I was going into my junior year. It would have been very difficult to do as a senior because of the seniors' tight schedule. The editorial duties were never a chore, but it was hard when we had both a test and a printer's deadline the next day. I never regretted the time spent on *Intervet,* because of all the wonderful people I had the chance to work with: student staff members, advisers, and busy veterinarians who wrote articles for us.

The cover and format of *Intervet* were changed while I was editor. The column "Viewpoints," my favorite feature in the journal, was developed to present the pros and cons on important issues such as animal rights versus animal welfare. We also included a national student survey about veterinary education in the first issue.

Nearly nine hundred students responded to the survey, and in general their responses supported many of the major changes in veterinary education that are being investigated by the Pew National Veterinary Education Program. A majority of the respondents favored specialized curriculum as a way to handle the problem of the increasing mass of veterinary information available to be taught, but most felt that a generalized curriculum should be offered concurrently. Subjects that a large percentage of students felt should receive more emphasis included business management, computer applications, alternate career pathways, and animal behavior.

Students are also concerned about state board

examinations. Some students believe that a D.V.M. degree should qualify you to practice anywhere in the United States. That's the way it is in Europe—once you graduate, you are not restricted to where you can practice. It's a difficult situation here, because each state requires an examination, and each state has different rules. Some states accept a higher or lower standard deviation on the National Board Exam, and others require a written or oral exam, as well as the national board and clinical competency tests. I know that regional differences exist, but I see state boards as an additional barrier for old or new graduates who might want to change locations.

I think this is an exciting time for veterinary medicine. In education and in other areas, things are changing. There is less satisfaction with traditional memorization-type education, which does nothing to stimulate creativity. We tend to memorize the names of muscles and bones for an exam and then forget the material immediately afterward. It's hard to see the importance of this information when it is not correlated with diseases or problems in animals. Most exams reward students who have raw mental-storage capacity. I'd like to see exams reward students who can take important information and apply it.

Classes need to be integrated. I think basic science classes could be spiced up with clinical cases. I enjoy clinics now that I am a senior. We get more hands-on experience, and I like taking information I have learned and turning it into something useful.

I have observed junior and senior students taking a special interest in different areas. Some of us will choose a specialty or research area based on that interest. I especially like surgery. I am not the best surgeon in the class, but neither am I the worst. I genuinely look forward to each surgery lab, overprepare for class, and do outside reading on procedures I am especially interested in.

I knew by my junior year in veterinary school that I wanted to concentrate on small-animal medicine. However, some students need a general curriculum. I think it's important to offer students options.

Tufts University School of Veterinary Medicine recently offered a trial surgical course, using cadavers instead of live animals, to third-year veterinary students who are opposed to vivisection. I think this is a viable option for students who plan to enter alternative careers, such as regulatory veterinary medicine or industry, that don't require surgical skills. However, I'm not sure that surgery on cadavers only is an acceptable substitute for someone who plans to enter veterinary practice. There's no question that dead tissue looks, feels, and behaves differently from live tissue, and students need to know how to handle the live tissue before performing procedures on animals that are of great emotional or monetary value to their owners. I think the Tufts plan allows for extra senior-year rotations in small-animal medicine and surgery to ensure live-tissue handling experience after students have trained on cadavers. This is just one example of the changes that are occurring in veterinary education.

Nine of ten members of the Students for the Alternative Program of Surgery, the Tufts student organization that petitioned for the new course, were women. I believe that many male students are also concerned with ethical issues such as this. However, sex-role stereotypes still exist that make it more difficult for men to be vocal about their feelings, or even to admit that they have strong feelings, about these issues. Conversely, a woman who advocates the use of animals in research may be more likely to be labeled insensitive than a man holding the same view. I think members of both sexes run the gamut in their opinions on controversial ethical issues, but conformity and societal expectations can influence the level of action we take based on those beliefs.

It's important for women to become involved in the issues and politics of our profession. One of the things I discovered as *Intervet* editor was that the people who are influential in the profession are nearly all male. The house of delegates to the American Veterinary Medical Association (AVMA) is 90 percent male. No woman has ever been AVMA president, and I don't know when women are going to break in. I hope that men in positions of power will act as mentors for women who aspire to AVMA political positions.

For women to break into positions of power, they are going to have to put some effort into it. It may take women who refuse to settle for the status quo, who are not afraid to make a fuss. I wrote about the topic of women in veterinary medicine in the January–February 1989 *Intervet* editorial:

> Interestingly, under current conditions, women who have the best chances of advancement may be those who enjoy, or even prefer, working with men. I'm not referring to the proverbial nail-filing coquette; in fact, I'm thinking of quite

the opposite—women who are competent, confident in their ability to succeed, and who view the traditionally male corporate politics not as a barrier but as a challenge, with their own fascinating set of stakes and rewards. When more women have joined the high ranks of the profession, the advantage will be to people of either gender who work well with people of either gender, which is what we ought to have been aiming for all along.

Women veterinarians are becoming more visible, and I think that will be positive for the profession as a whole. Debbye Turner, a senior veterinary student at the University of Missouri, was named Miss America in 1990. I think it's to the pageant's credit that it chose a woman as academically oriented and career-minded as she is. Her reign will remind the public that veterinary medicine is no longer a field for males only and that women are making unique and important contributions to the profession.

I believe veterinary medicine is a great career for men or women, and in spite of pessimistic forecasts about the job market and salaries, I am optimistic about the future. I believe that if you really want something, there's always something out there for you. Your first job may not be exactly what you want or where you want to go, but if you start somewhere, you'll eventually get to where you want to be. For instance, a new graduate who wants to specialize in small animals might have to start out in a mixed-animal practice.

I think my classmates and I have realistic expectations. Most of my classmates expect to go into a practice and live in a nice area. In the long run, if you are only in something for the money, you will burn out. I want to feel like I've accomplished something or helped someone at the end of the workday. One of the best feelings I remember was in the practice in England. I went into the exam room to see a dog I had helped perform surgery on the week before. The dog was happy and wagging its tail. That's deeper than money.

One of the good things that has come out of the tighter job market is that veterinarians have begun looking at careers outside of practice and have made a place for themselves in nontraditional jobs using their veterinary training. I like the fact that there are so many rooms in a big building. There are many options, and I feel that I can make a career change within the profession if I like.

Of course, it might narrow my choices later on if I were married. I'm at a point now where I'm very protective of my freedom. There are so many things I want to do before I'm tied down with a family. It's also exhausting just getting through my schedule as it is now. It would be a lot harder married. My classmate Jackie Piepkorn, who shares emergency duty with me tonight, is married and has a one-year-old boy. Jackie is the kind of organized person who can handle numerous obligations, but it must be hard.

A lot of my friends and classmates have married veterinarians, but the majority have married professionals in other fields. I want to be married and have a family someday, but it would take someone who would give me a lot of freedom and would want an independent life-style for both of us.

I want to obtain experience in small-animal practice right after school. I would also like to locate, at least for a while, in Minneapolis to be closer to Mom. I've always enjoyed academics, so I know that at some point I might go back to school for an internship or a residency. Plus, I've grown accustomed to living in university towns, which offer cultural events and stimulating classes. I also hope to continue with my writing, both free-lance writing for professional journals and creative writing. All of these factors will affect my decision about jobs after graduation.

In any case, I know I'll find an area or many areas of veterinary medicine that I love. If you work at what you love, you will always give forth your best effort, and the rewards will be many. I can't wait to get started. ∎

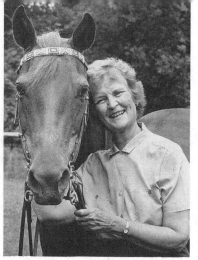

photo by Jack Foley

Elizabeth Atwood Lawrence

COMBINING two major disciplines— veterinary medicine and anthropology— Elizabeth Atwood Lawrence emerged as the first veterinary anthropologist. As such, she studies animals' roles in past and present cultures, and concludes that technology places humans' relationship with animals and the natural world in grave trouble. All her enthusiasm and dedication are now focused on under- standing and improving the human- animal relationship.

"Knowledge of this relationship is fundamental to the veterinary pro- fession," she says. "In the past, researchers have often viewed animals only from the human perspective, focusing on their use and exploitation. I strive to give the animals' own input the full, scholarly, analytical study it deserves."

Believing that marriage and children are equally as important as a career, Lawrence found the strength and stamina to succeed at both. For fifteen years she operated her own veterinary practice while raising her son and

daughter, instilling in them her love of animals and nature. When her children were in elementary school, Lawrence, who had obtained her doctor of veterinary medicine degree in 1956 from the University of Pennsylvania, returned to graduate school and earned a master of arts degree in cultural anthropology from Brown University. Her 1976 thesis, "Centaurs of the Plains: The Horse in Crow Indian Culture, Past and Present," won the Elsie Clews Parsons Award of the American Ethnological Society. In 1979 she received her Ph.D. degree. Her doctoral dissertation, on rodeos, won the 1980 James Moody Award of the Southern Anthropological Society.

Living among the Crow Indians of Montana for a summer and frequenting western rodeos for several years, Lawrence found that animals are a communicating bond. From those experiences as well as many other studies, Lawrence authored three books: *Rodeo: An Anthropologist Looks at the Wild and the Tame* (1982), *Hoofbeats and Society: Studies of Human-Horse*

Interactions (1985), and *His Very Silence Speaks: Comanche—The Horse Who Survived Custer's Last Stand* (1989). *Rodeo* is now required reading in many courses ranging from American culture to wildlife conservation at such universities as Harvard, Cornell, the University of California at San Diego, the University of North Carolina, and the University of Calgary. Recently, in appreciation of her work, Lawrence was named to membership in the Western Writers of America.

In 1981 Lawrence was appointed to a full-time position on the faculty of the Tufts University School of Veterinary Medicine, with duties in both teaching and research. There she continued her pioneer endeavor, begun at Brown, to create and teach the first required course on human-animal relationships for veterinary students. She is now an associate professor in the school's Department of Environmental Studies.

"Every year, in the minds of seventy-two or more veterinary students at Tufts, I instill concepts, old and new, about human-animal interactions and about the significance of these interactions to their future professional careers," Lawrence says. "As veterinarians, they will take these ideas and spread them to clients and groups in their communities. Helping the students to become better informed and more compassionate veterinarians is the most significant part of my work."

Presently the foremost educator and authority nationally and internationally on the human relationship to animals and the natural environment, Lawrence received the first International Distinguished Scholar Award from the Delta Society in 1989, at the Fifth International Conference on Relationships between Humans and Animals.

Prominent at a time when the urgency of preserving animals and nature is a vital worldwide concern, Lawrence is fully aware of the need for solutions. Her twenty-nine-page curriculum vitae records awards and accomplishments achieved since beginning her career in veterinary anthropology. Among them are the Bustad Companion Animal Veterinarian of the Year Award for the state of Massachusetts (1987), the Association for Women Veterinarians Outstanding Woman Veterinarian of the Year Award (1988), and the Mount Holyoke College Sesquicentennial Award (1988). Her writings appear in many refereed scholarly journals and as chapters in books. She is in constant demand as a speaker and has appeared on radio and television, including a 1983 TV program, "Who Needs Nature?" produced by the Canadian Broadcasting Company. Publishers frequently seek her expertise in reviewing manuscripts, articles, and books.

Lawrence harmonizes well with the fields and woods of Westport, Massachusetts, where her home is hidden among the trees just a few miles from the ocean. Golden Dream Farm is her forest primeval, where nature rules undisturbed, providing peace and serenity.

"Why is it that people will not cherish and protect our wilderness until they see the wild shrinking and innumerable species being lost?" Lawrence asks. "Adults must encourage a sense of wonder in children for each creature's special abilities and its value within the ecosystem. Earth has been greatly damaged, but now there is a movement toward a more appreciative view in which people think, 'Let each creature live, and let's try to get along with it.' I'm doing all I can to encourage this attitude."

From the first moment I can remember, I felt
a great love for animals. When I was very young, I had a black-and-
white cat named Skeezix, who would follow me on walks. At four,
I saw my first horse and was infected with an intense case of
horseitis, so that for years I begged for a horse. I was a city child,
born in Boston and raised in Fall River, Massachusetts, but my
parents managed to satisfy this tremendous desire when I was
sixteen. Once I had my own horse, I spent every possible minute
riding and caring for it, as though to make up for the time lost in
waiting. My father always understood my deep need for a horse. He
encouraged me to become an expert rider and showed his pride in
my accomplishments by taking many photographs and movies of
me with my horse.

Despite my animal involvement, my interests were always
well rounded. I wrote poetry as a child and won prizes for my poetry
in high school. One of my poems was about the power of thought and
how people can think themselves to faraway places. Another
featured the beauty and skill of my father's hands, because he was
a surgeon. I wrote a poem for each of my pets, but horses always
inspired the most poetry. I loved philosophy and social science, as
well as biology, and read everything I could find involving human
relationships with animals.

My father, an obstetrician and surgeon who was totally
dedicated to his patients, still found time to spend with me. He often
read medical poetry to me, and I learned early that my scholarly
efforts didn't have to be compartmentalized. Science and the
humanities, medicine, and classic literature and poetry could all be
studied. All my life I have had a great love for books.

My father encouraged me to be a veterinarian. He believed
in the concept of one medicine, finding nobility in the healing art
used either for human or animal. This was an unusual attitude
then and even now. His colleagues would say, "You must make your
daughter become a physician," because they believed human beings
were at the center of the universe. Animals had no value except to
make a better life for people. Medical doctors often have an
anthropocentric view.

My mother did not have a career and had difficulty
understanding why I wanted to be a veterinarian. She thought all
women should be wives and mothers. I was probably part of the last
generation of women who were discouraged from making a career.
But my father urged me to ignore the demands of that social
custom. He saw no barriers for women. He felt that, like men,

women were limited only by their desires and abilities. He called me his "horse doctor" with great affection and respect.

My father introduced me to the joys of nature study. Recently, I wrote an article about wild birds as therapy for human patients and dedicated it to him. Fifty years ago he realized how important nature was to healing people. One of his patients was a young doctor with tuberculosis. In those days tuberculosis patients were secluded in a sanatorium for months or years of rest. This man was very depressed about interrupting his medical career, so my father sent him binoculars and a bird identification book. Delighted by his observations of different birds, each beautiful in flight, he forgot his own problems and made a good recovery. When I talk to that doctor today, he recalls how much bird-watching meant to him. Using animals for therapy is now an accepted practice, but my father was way ahead of his time.

I went to Mount Holyoke College, an intellectually challenging all-women's college in South Hadley, Massachusetts. Without men, women were bolder in class discussion and competed for responsible positions like class president and newspaper editor, usually reserved for men. Young women acquired a sense of self-worth at Mount Holyoke, and many were determined to follow a career. Though others have since followed me, I was the first graduate to become a veterinarian. The education I received at Mount Holyoke was a very important preparation for the difficulties a woman encountered at that time in entering a male-dominated profession.

When the University of Pennsylvania veterinary school accepted me, I felt privileged. If society was willing to allow me to be a veterinarian, I would try to be perfect in every way—an outstanding veterinarian and scholar as well as the best possible wife and mother. At that time many women felt obligated to fill all their roles well. That was certainly more of a burden than any human being should carry.

I entered veterinary school with a liberal arts degree and an English major, a very unusual background in those days. I credit my undergraduate study of humanities with sharpening my sensitivity to the joy and beauty of animals and nature and with helping me gain an understanding of human-animal interactions. Today at Tufts, more of the veterinary students have liberal arts degrees.

When I attended veterinary school, Pennsylvania admitted an even number of women, either two or four, so they could be partners in the clinics. The faculty and male students felt that a woman wasted a man's space in the school because she would never practice. I did not fulfill that unjustified prophecy and even treated my patients right up until the morning I gave birth to my daughter.

Back then, women students were denied full participation at the veterinary school. We were excluded from the students' room, where men relaxed and where exam schedules and notices were posted, and we were not allowed to join the veterinary fraternity. During my first year, I roomed with a senior student whose schedule sounded wonderful. She rode for four weeks on farm calls, accompanying four different large-animal clinicians. Because in my future practice I planned to treat horses, I knew the value of such experience. Looking forward to gaining that practical knowledge of farm-animal medicine helped me to endure the hard courses during the first three years.

At the start of my final year, I rushed with great anticipation to the veterinary school to find my schedule. To my horror, women had been eliminated from the ambulatory practice rotations. Overcoming my natural reticence, I met with the dean to argue for the women students' participation in those four weeks. One of the reasons for our exclusion, he told me, was that the clinicians' wives had complained about women students accompanying their husbands on calls. I could not believe that such mistrustful wives had that kind of power over my career. Finally, through my efforts, the dean allowed one week with a practitioner for each woman in the class.

A Saturday field trip once took my class to the famous Hanover Shoe Farm, a trotting-horse farm in Pennsylvania. There, at the start of our tour, the women were told that they would not be allowed to accompany the rest of the class into the breeding barn. I couldn't believe this was happening. Although there was no activity in the barn at the time, an old taboo still excluded women from even setting foot in that area.

I wanted to be a veterinarian with such intensity that I could endure anything to meet that goal. The men, by comparison, took their education for granted. Even the all-male faculty were not wise enough to recognize or empathize with my dedication and recognize my potential contribution. Sexist attitudes were prevalent. But these prejudices never killed my enthusiasm.

In those days, veterinary school was regimented, somewhat like an army camp. The faculty owed little respect to the students. Teachers could behave inappropriately and belittle the students without fear of rebellion. Today students have a great deal of power. They make demands, and the professors comply. There should be a happy medium between these two states.

Between my third and fourth years of veterinary school, students were required to work for a veterinarian during the summer. I wrote many letters seeking a job, but only one small-animal doctor agreed to hire me. For six weeks he treated me like an outsider. He didn't allow me to be present when he was talking to clients or explaining his diagnoses. In contrast, I remembered how my father felt an instant affinity with anyone wanting to be a physician, and I couldn't understand this difference in attitude.

Women were treated with inequality in veterinary school, but we still excelled. My senior friend won top scholastic honors at graduation. I ranked high in my class and was elected to membership in Phi Zeta, the honor society of veterinary medicine.

In those days, many people perceived veterinarians as they were portrayed in the movies: as unshaven drunks who frequented dark smelly barns—vulgar places definitely off-limits for sensitive women. In media presentations, often a medical doctor was called in to treat a particularly important or valuable animal. Some of my childhood acquaintances were horrified when they heard I was studying to be a veterinarian. In my veterinary school yearbook, I'm characterized as a "rare china cup in a bull pen."

After graduation, I decided to take Florida's state board exam. My interest in Florida wildlife was strong, and I had relatives there. The faculty and some of my classmates told me I could pass only if I had professional contacts in that state. But I succeeded without them. I am licensed to practice in five states.

I still remember my first job offer. A veterinarian near my home in Massachusetts interviewed me, and we got along well. He told me to start working for him in two weeks. I arrived in my white coat, with my new stethoscope, flushed with excitement. His wife met me at the door. "My husband has changed his mind," she said. Again my tremendous enthusiasm made me vulnerable.

Following that, I worked at two Massachusetts small-animal hospitals where a replacement veterinarian was needed. During that time, I met my husband, Robert Lawrence, who was the assistant minister of my church. When my grandmother died, the senior minister was on vacation, so Bob handled her funeral. That was in the fall, and in June, a year after my graduation, we were married—a quiet young veterinarian and a gregarious minister.

Because I already had my career when my husband married me, he found it quite agreeable to have a veterinarian for a wife. Sometimes when a woman pursues a career later in marriage, her husband may feel cheated of time and attention.

Bob and I wanted to explore the West, so Bob accepted a job as prison chaplain at Terminal Island, and we lived in Long Beach, California. On our days off, we camped in our station wagon, traveling up and down the coast and visiting many national parks and monuments. We were able to see many new birds and wild animals during these trips.

I couldn't practice without a license, and while I waited to take the California state board exam, I worked for the National Audubon Society in El Monte, teaching natural history and conservation to children, grade school through junior high. I remember that the director of the Audubon center had several tame tarantulas, and she let one of the giant hairy creatures crawl on her arm while I explained their amazing, yet harmless abilities. Children who previously thought all tarantulas should be smashed with a rock were suddenly enthralled by their gentleness.

At about the same time, I answered an ad in a veterinary journal for a writer-editor. "That's for me," I thought. "I have a degree in English, training in writing, and a veterinary degree." The reply letter told me I was the best-qualified applicant, but considerable travel, the employers felt, made the job unsuitable for a woman. A woman, they indicated, belonged at home with her husband. In those days, sex was a legal basis for rejection.

Once licensed in California, I practiced companion-animal medicine with several different veterinarians and gained a great deal of experience. After three years on the West Coast, we returned to Westport, Massachusetts, where I built my animal hospital. In my own practice, I never encountered sexist attitudes. People knew me and consulted me because they wanted a woman. One client kept beautiful Guernsey cows and talked to them as though they were sensitive, perceptive ladies. I was the only veterinarian chosen to treat his "girls." He considered men too rough. Most of my practice consisted of companion animals and horses, but I enjoyed treating a few sheep and cows and many injured wild birds.

In 1964 my daughter, Priscilla, was born, and two years later my son, Mark. I hired a woman to care for them, but my animal hospital was only a short distance from the house, so I could dash in and see them whenever there was a lull in my schedule.

Bob had his own church and frequently worked at night. In

the daytime he could come home if the children needed him. Every morning and whenever there were emergencies, he helped me in the animal hospital and went on farm calls with me. As the children grew, they also assisted in the animal hospital. My work greatly expanded their world. They saw puppies and kittens born naturally and by cesarian section. Surrounded by a positive aura of healing, both children loved animals. This interest extended to nature, and Bob and I took the children on camping trips during the summer and on many hikes in the woods and along the seashore. My work was never like a job; it was a labor of love. I worked on many weekends and holidays and after hours. But though my profession took much of my time, our children were always a top priority. Children have to know they're loved and that they're important, or they won't develop into the kind of people that parents want them to be. Bob and I always went to their school plays and tried to be present for all significant occasions. When my daughter was in college at Mount Holyoke, and when my son was majoring in history at Stanford, I often read the same books they were reading and discussed their ideas. We continue to do this.

The children were five and seven when I bought a Morgan mare who was in foal. Today we still have the same mare and her son, a chestnut gelding. Priscilla often rides with me, and sometimes Mark rides too. Priscilla earned a master's degree in social science at the University of Chicago and is now in her final year at Yale Divinity School, studying to be a minister. She says she gets many of her ideas about healing from me, but she wants to work with people. She took an environmental ethics course at Yale that attempts to incorporate into the Judeo-Christian religions the positive message that God gives human beings an obligation to preserve nature and its species. This is what Priscilla believes and will teach as part of her ministry. Mark has just earned his master's degree in history from Stanford. He plans to work for a couple of years before he begins studying for his Ph.D. He enjoys journalism, and during his undergraduate years he was a reporter for the Stanford University newspaper and became its editor. He has had internships with the *Washington Post* and the *New York Times* and is presently a research assistant for NATO in Belgium. My children share many of my interests, especially those I never had the opportunity to develop.

During the seventies, I returned to Brown University to study anthropology and gradually eased out of veterinary practice. I was motivated by my desire to study human-animal relationships on a deep level and to obtain scholarly theoretical training that would allow me to carry out research that would contribute substantially to this field. During my years of graduate study, I remember parking my car pointing toward home so that I could rush from my last class to meet my children at the school bus. After school is such an important time to be with children; there is a flow of conversation that might never happen again.

Since my days in college and veterinary school, there has been a kind of social revolution. In the fifties, undergraduate life was dignified and conservative. No liquor was allowed on campus. When a student's father carried her suitcases into the dormitory, she called out "Man coming," and all the women would disappear. Now boyfriends stay overnight in women's rooms. I was amazed at the dress and language of the seventies on campus, which were so different. Adults have to be good sports to adjust to such radical changes.

At Brown, even though I had not written a research paper for more than twenty years, I had no trouble with the class work. I loved learning, and reading the assigned books was pure joy. Some professors at Brown saw me not as a professional person but as the stereotype of an older woman who returned to college after raising children. Because I had shouldered the responsibilities of doctoring animals and managing my own veterinary hospital for many years, I felt strongly I was not in that category.

I had to convince professors that it was possible to combine veterinary medicine and anthropology. For my master's and Ph.D. degrees I completed twenty-four courses—a lot of courses on top of foreign-language requirements, fieldwork, and a thesis and a dissertation. Some of the classes I shaped myself, adding new dimensions of animal-behavior observations to anthropology. Anthropologists had often viewed animals mainly as symbols in human cognition or as tools in cultural change, but I wanted to include in my studies the dimensions of the living animal as it interacts with people. Several professors saw the potential of my work in human-animal relationships and provided encouragement.

Whereas students in most academic disciplines can do their research in the library, anthropology students go to live with people in various societies and cultures. For my fieldwork, I chose western rodeos because human-animal relationships are its center. Because I was raised in the East, the West was like a foreign culture. I wanted to fully understand rodeos, so in addition to anthropology courses, I took courses on the history and theory of performance and the history and meaning of the American frontier. Cowboy life contrasted so sharply with my own eastern values, it made the ranch-rodeo society stand out in bold relief. I analyzed and wrote about customs and ideas that westerners take for granted.

Armed with a letter from Brown explaining my credentials, I approached the Professional Rodeo Cowboys Association. I sought permission to wander freely behind the scenes at sanctioned rodeos throughout the American Great Plains.

As I explained in my book, "Rodeos provide valuable information about the ways people perceive of and participate in relationships with animals and also with nature and the wild. On a deeper level rodeo offers insights into the manner in which a given socio-cultural group may deal with the universal dilemma of man's place in nature. Rodeo . . . is not only stating what the West was and is but what the present society wishes it to continue to be."

While I waited for a decision from the rodeo cowboys association, I attended nonsanctioned rodeos for contrast. I spent a whole week at the Women's Rodeo Championship Finals, which gave me many insights, and went to several Little Britches (children's) rodeos. I even talked to participants in an eastern rodeo who had no background in ranching.

The Professional Rodeo Cowboys Association finally interviewed me to find out how I planned to use my information. In the past a few easterners had focused on cruelty in rodeos. The cowboys felt that untruths were told, and rodeos were harmed. Even the *New York Times* has printed an inaccurate statement in an ad indicating that rodeo cowboys placed tacks under their saddles. Unfortunately, there is cruelty wherever horses and animals are used in sport or entertainment, as in horse shows and racing as well as rodeos, but that was not the special focus of my study.

During my fieldwork on the Great Plains ranch-rodeo complex, I followed the western rodeo circuit, including the famous Calgary Stampede and Cheyenne Frontier Days. I interviewed individual cowboys, trying to capture their perceptions, feelings, and cultural attitudes. My empathy and interest in them made me a good listener. A skillful interviewer does not interrupt or dominate the conversation.

Most aspects of traditional cowboy culture generally exclude women. My press pass allowed me into the chute area, where I was often the only female. Stiff and wary of me at first, the cowboys soon treated me with great chivalry and were careful not to swear in front of me. I wore western dress and showed respect for their customs. There were a few tense moments. In that brawling, chaotic environment I may have seemed comically out of place, climbing on the chutes while juggling my camera, notebook, and pen. I was successful, however, because the cowboys loved talking about horses and bulls and other rodeo animals, and so they relaxed in my presence.

Rodeo first caught my attention in the summer of 1975 when I was in Montana studying the significance of the horse among the Crow Indians for my master's thesis. There I saw my first Indian rodeo, in which the Crows and several visiting tribes participated with enthusiasm. I had been warned that American Indians had been overstudied and were unfriendly to intrusive anthropologists. But I had no trouble when I said, "I'm here to study horses." The Crows love their horses and knew that I shared their feelings.

Societies like the Plains Indians lived in harmony with their environment and had an interdependence with nature. Their myths and legends, their religion and worldview, reflect the beauty and importance of nature. Many of them visualize life as a circle in which each creature occupies its own niche as an important part of the whole and shares equally with humankind. I am fascinated by their legends that describe animals giving gifts of knowledge to human beings, imparting special wisdom to enable people to survive in the wilderness. The Cheyenne even tell stories about animals helping God create the earth, with humans and animals working together. In contrast, the Judeo-Christian religion views life as a ladder or hierarchy with God at the top, then angels, then humankind, and below them, the animals, ranked in importance, with primates and mammals high, insects low. If our variety of animals and plants is to be preserved, we must teach children that *dominion* in Genesis really means *stewardship*. Humans are obligated to respect, care for, and conserve the animals. Children must learn that animals have their own value. What is a snake good for? Sure, it is useful in controlling other species we call pests. But children must also realize that a snake has its own place in the world and a right to live.

As an associate professor in the Department of Environmental Studies at Tufts University School of Veterinary Medicine, I teach first-year veterinary students a required course in human-animal relationships. This is an innovative course, the only one of its kind. When I designed the course, I had to compromise between what I'd like the students to know and what the students see as directly related to their career in veterinary medicine. Veterinary students tend to be very pragmatic. But the parameters of the profession are constantly expanding, and so the course combines social science and other disciplines with veterinary medicine. In place of a textbook, I assign readings in books and journals. I find informed speakers to present their views on many subjects. Some topics, like animal welfare and animal rights, are controversial, and I am very careful to present all sides of those issues. My students listen, question, and come to their own conclusions. Amidst the first-year curriculum's demands for scientific fact and memorization, my course provides an oasis of thought, and students tell me they rediscover their motivation for becoming veterinarians.

First I provide background information on people and concepts involved in human-animal relationships, past and present. This orients students to the issues of the course. One speaker explains why Americans prefer certain kinds of animals and what factors affect public attitudes toward wildlife and conservation. We explore the idea that animals are able to help people heal mentally and physically. Domestication brings with it new diseases and behavior problems, so we discuss its effect. We study the social structure of the wild antecedents of domestic animals and the changing role of zoos. We also discuss the differences between people and animals and the question of human uniqueness.

Human-animal relationships is a much broader topic than the human-animal bond. The latter usually refers to health benefits for people: animals helping the handicapped in hospitals, the elderly in nursing homes, or lonely people in institutions or at home. Animals do seem to restore human health, but this is hard to prove to people who demand scientific data. We cover the significance of pets in American society and issues related to euthanasia, pet death, and client bereavement. We study both sides of the question of the use of animals in research. We probe for answers to why our society is so destructive toward wildlife. These topics are very important for contemporary veterinarians. I stay after class for students who want to discuss the subjects further. A majority of veterinary students now come from the city. Sometimes they have to be taught how to handle livestock, yet they are often more sensitive to animals' feelings than students with rural backgrounds. On the farm, where animals are raised for profit to be slaughtered, a more utilitarian view develops. Both groups thank me for encouraging their desire to help animals.

My time is divided between teaching, research, and writing. My position at Tufts from the beginning specified that, because of my unique background and training, I would spend my time carrying out field research and writing whenever I am not on campus for teaching, meeting with students, or working on committees, or away speaking at conferences. Firsthand studies that involve interviewing people are very important to my work in veterinary anthropology. When I studied the mounted police in Boston for my book *Hoofbeats and Society,* for example, I talked to the police officers themselves and also interviewed people on the street to discover what feelings a police officer on a horse stirred in them. Studies show that in the presence of an animal people are more friendly and talk more freely. Some so-called hard scientists believe that thought and feeling have no valid meaning. But the interview technique actually provides highly significant information. When researchers in any scholarly discipline filter data through their minds, their conclusions are colored by personal interpretation. Margaret Mead's Samoa, for instance, was very different from a more recent account by another anthropologist. Both can be accurate in their observations. Experienced at different times, cultures can change, and resulting data vary with the approach of the particular field-worker.

My book on the horse Comanche has just been published. In 1958 I was at the battlefield of the Little Bighorn in Montana when I learned that a horse survived Custer's last stand. I was so anxious to learn more about this horse that my husband and I drove nonstop to see Comanche, who is mounted as a museum exhibit at the University of Kansas in Lawrence. It took a long time and a great deal of effort to collect and document all of this celebrated horse's history and lore, but my enthusiasm never waned. The life and legend of Comanche sheds much light on the role of animals in society and the symbolic meaning they embody. Doing research and writing books is very demanding and requires a great many sacrifices, but I find it extremely rewarding. I have ideas that I'm really excited about for more books and am anxious to get started.

My love and appreciation for animals and nature only became deeper with time. Humankind's aesthetic being and even our very existence are tied to preserving the widest possible variety of plants and animals. The elephant, the gorilla, and the rain forests hold many secrets people have yet to discover. The elephant is very intelligent, with many remarkable abilities, and people must realize that it is wrong to destroy such an extraordinary creature. Americans' appetite for cheap beef, now spreading throughout the world, encourages South Americans to transform rain forests into grazing land for cattle. Habitat destruction is rapidly depleting many species. The beautiful scarlet tanager declines with the rain forests that are its winter range. I'm convinced we must sacrifice comforts and financial gains to save our wilderness, but how do we teach people to be less materialistic? Children are influenced by the way adults react to animals. Once I saw some youngsters pulling the wings off insects. Other adults watching them said, "That's what children do. They all go through that stage, and you can't stop them." But my children never tried to hurt any living thing. They were kind to all creatures through example. Education is also an important key to saving the animals. It is fortunate that some nature conservation groups are setting up programs to dispense vital information, especially in schools.

Cross-cultural studies also have much to teach about attitudes toward animals and the conservation of animals and nature. I've learned a great deal from studying the ranch-rodeo complex. Dating from the time of the cattle frontier, there has been an antagonism toward the wild that exists simultaneously with an admiration for it. This ambivalent attitude has been a strong factor in determining American interaction with nature and animals. When you make a very careful in-depth scholarly study of one society's relationships to animals, principles may emerge that can be successfully applied to other groups and situations. For example, I have been very gratified to hear from an eminent animal behaviorist and ecologist that my rodeo data helped him understand the people he deals with in his work in wildlife conservation. As a result, he uses my book as a text in the course he gives for students who will enter this field.

Many species are becoming extinct. The last of the California condors are now in a zoo, where attendants remove eggs from the female's clutch so that she is stimulated to lay more eggs. The hatchlings are fed by puppets made to look like adult condors so the young birds do not imprint on humans. Animals must not be allowed to bond to people if they are to be successful in returning to the wild. The central role of zoos has changed from entertainment and fun to serious attempts at breeding vanishing species to restock their natural environment. To reprogram an animal to feed and protect itself in the wild is very difficult and time-consuming, and success has been limited. Even so, we must continue to try. This process is the only hope for some species. But to make it work, of course, habitats must also be preserved. The condors' range must be kept free of development so the birds can be returned to it in the future.

In 1981 I made contact with the Masai tribe of Africa. I'm fascinated by these herders who live so close to their cattle in what has been called a symbiotic relationship. Their songs and poetry revolve around their cattle, which are an intermediary between the Masai and God. People drink milk and sometimes the blood, but they kill and eat the cattle only as part of a special ritual. Their standard greeting is "I hope your cattle are well."

Regarding the so-called feminization of the veterinary profession, we don't know what effects it may have. A study carried out by Dr. Steve Kellert from Yale sampled the general American population and concluded that women are more interested than men in humane issues. Women's feeling for individual animals is more emotional and sentimental than the men's. We can't as yet conclude that the increase of women in veterinary medicine will make the profession more oriented toward animal welfare and animal rights. This has not been proven. Women who choose veterinary medicine may not think the way women in the rest of the population do.

Anthropology is a field in which women are accepted, and I've always felt veterinary medicine is a natural career for women because it involves a great deal of nurturance. But society for a long time denied this connection. Anthropology also requires so-called feminine qualities like the ability to listen to people and empathize with them, and the adaptability required to live harmoniously among people with different customs.

Today there is a new, more subtle kind of sexism operating in many spheres as well as in veterinary medicine. Women are accepted in school and in practice. When it comes to providing opportunities for holding offices and obtaining prestigious positions and promotions, men in charge are apt to favor women who are not married or those they consider not feminine. The women who advance are likely to be those who are perceived as totally committed to their careers, like the traditional men. Sexism shows sometimes when my male colleagues talk to me about personal details rather than my research. Middle-aged and older men have been raised to see a woman as a female first and then a professional person. Fortunately, this is changing in younger men.

For a number of years, I served on the admissions committee

at Tufts. When I interviewed a woman who was extremely bright, enthusiastic, and well educated, I thought, "What a wonderful veterinarian you'll make!" Then I would realize that in the old days, a man who was just average would have been accepted in her place.

In anthropology, my female colleagues were often less friendly after I won awards for my writing and began to be recognized in their field. Many women are competitive and haven't learned to help one another. Women veterinarians who had to fight for acceptance should be willing to extend a helping hand to those who are just beginning. In veterinary medicine, we must remember that full equality for women has not yet been achieved. Positions of authority and power are still generally reserved for men. Females will soon become the majority in the profession, though, and this gives them the opportunity to influence the profession in a positive way. I'm hoping we will create our own dimensions, enhance our nurturing role. The world of living things badly needs protection and kindness.

My career is developing very rapidly. I work at it all the time because it is what I love to do. As Robert Frost phrased it in his poem "Two Tramps in Mud Time," I am able to "unite my avocation and my vocation." There is so much I want to accomplish that the days are not long enough. Every day I get new ideas about human-animal relationships that I want to study and write about. The mail brings invitations for me to speak at conferences or write articles. I've even been asked to sign a contract ahead of time for my next book. I'm very pleased to be able to make my contributions to deepen our understanding of human interactions with animals and with the natural world. Knowledge in this field is urgently needed today if we are to counteract the terrible human destructiveness that characterizes our ecological crisis and are to save not only other species but ourselves as well. My teaching is particularly important because I have the opportunity to present my veterinary students with new and relevant concepts regarding human-animal relationships and to motivate them to meet the challenges that lie ahead in creating a better world for both animals and people. ■

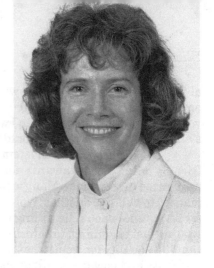

Sandra V. McNeel

SANDRA V. McNEEL is a board-certified veterinary radiologist. While serving as head of the radiology section at the Veterinary Teaching Hospital at Iowa State University, McNeel taught veterinary students, served on national and university committees, wrote journal articles and chapters of radiology texts, and made presentations at national conventions. McNeel was honored as one of the Outstanding Young Women of America in 1979 and received the Amoco Outstanding Teacher Award in the College of Veterinary Medicine (Iowa State University) in 1986.

Electing to leave her successful academic career behind, McNeel recently embarked in a new direction. Her plans at the time she was interviewed for this book included selling her home in Iowa, moving to California, and accepting a temporary six-month term as a radiologist at the University of California. McNeel described the unknown in her future as frightening, but she also spoke with a sense of relief and anticipation.

Although McNeel pictures herself as a left-brain-oriented scientist, she desires to develop her creative, or right-brain, talents. She foresees a professional career that will allow free time to participate in her hobby: dancing and singing in theater productions. With light-brown hair and twinkling eyes, McNeel appears younger than her age, and it's easy to visualize her in costume for "Annie Get Your Gun" or "Oklahoma!"

■

I was raised in the San Fernando Valley, a metropolitan area of Los Angeles. My grandfather owned a company that brought prime beef in from the Midwest and fabricated it for the restaurant and hotel trade in L.A. My dad worked for the company in a sort of mid-management position, and my mom was a traditional homemaker.

I have one sister who is a couple of years younger than I. We are very close but have always been on the opposite end of things. My sister is very right-brained—creative and artistic. Although I participated in theater productions in high school, my interests at that time were more scientific. I finally decided as a twelve- or thirteen-year-old that becoming a cowgirl was economically unfeasible, and I changed my aspirations to veterinary medicine.

My parents were encouraging about my desire to become a veterinarian. We had many pets, primarily dogs because my dad was anti-cat, and I enjoyed the animals. When I was a teenager, I worked several consecutive summers at a local small-animal hospital. By the time I graduated from high school, my goal to become a veterinarian was well defined.

I wrote to several veterinary schools and received a list of preprofessional requirements. I chose Colorado State University because it sounded more exciting than central California, where I was raised. Every third person on campus seemed to be in preveterinary medicine, and we got together to share notes, study, and go on ski trips. I met some great people and look back on those two years at CSU as some of the good times.

After I finished my sophomore year, I applied to veterinary schools in Colorado, Washington, and California. I received a letter from each one of them that read "Our sincere regrets . . ." The letter from Colorado was a form letter with a little note on the bottom informing me that Colorado accepted only residents or students from states that had contracts with CSU. It was obvious that I had no chance of getting into any school except in California, my resident state.

I decided that it would be to my advantage to complete my third year of preprofessional studies at the University of California at Davis. When I applied to veterinary school at the end of that year, I was accepted.

I started veterinary school at UC in 1968 as one of eight women in a class of eighty-two freshmen. I wasn't aware of any biases against women students by classmates or faculty. Because the women were always in the upper 10 percent of the class in scholastic achievement, our male classmates may have felt competitive in that area; however, for the most part, we felt a lot of camaraderie for each other. Of course, you could always count on a few professors to offer a couple of crude jokes or slip in a slide of bare-chested women. Today that would be considered inappropriate, but in those days we considered it part of being one of the guys. I enjoyed being one of the fellows and having all those brothers.

There seemed to be a preconceived idea, especially among women outside of veterinary school, that women in veterinary school were there to find husbands. I didn't want to be involved in anything that smacked of being there to get a husband.

Veterinary students did everything together, and it was hard to form social or dating relationships outside of veterinary school. My first concept was to avoid personal relationships with men in my class. For one thing, if the relationship waned, there was no way of avoiding the other party. Regardless of my resolve on the subject, I didn't quite make it.

It was during veterinary school that I recognized the time commitment that was required for my career. I thought that I would have difficulty combining career and marriage. That is the way we thought in those days. Very few women who went to veterinary school were married. Today many veterinary students, both male and female, are married, have children, and have children while in veterinary school. To have become pregnant while in veterinary school would have been asking to be booted out when I was a student. To put anything above veterinary medicine was considered sinful.

Most faculty members now realize that the best veterinarians are not necessarily produced by cramming an overwhelming number of facts into students' heads before they escape the process. A well-rounded individual who has knowledge in other areas and who has time to interact with a family is usually a happier and better-adjusted veterinarian.

When I was in veterinary school, women were just beginning to fill junior clinical faculty positions in professional schools. I remember that I admired Dr. Denise Colgrove, one of our clinicians, because of her caring attitude toward students and patients. I hoped that I would do as well. At that time I anticipated becoming a small-animal practitioner. In my opinion, teaching ranked low, just above meat inspection, as an area of interest.

The closer I got to graduation, the more I panicked and thought that I didn't know enough. I decided that, for my own professional development as well as my confidence, I would pursue an internship. I picked out several veterinary schools and large hospitals, such as Animal Medical Center (AMC) in New York and applied for internships in small-animal medicine. I was offered a position in AMC's cardiovascular section, but I turned it down because it appeared to be research-oriented, and I wanted clinical medicine. As it turned out, I had no job at graduation.

Soon after graduation, Dr. Chuck Farrow, a classmate who had an internship at Oklahoma State University, called and told me that the small-animal department had added a slot for another intern. I figured I could stand anything for a year, so I accepted an internship at OSU. It was there that I got my first experience with teaching.

Chuck and I had very good backgrounds in clinical radiology, and I had completed an elective rotation in radiology at the University of California. The OSU veterinary students noticed that we seemed to know what we were doing when it came to interpreting radiographs. Several students were interested in learning our techniques, so Chuck and I started an informal after-hours radiology course. Those bright students had such interest and desire to learn, and Chuck and I had a great time instructing them.

As the only interns in small-animal medicine and surgery, Chuck and I rotated taking small-animal emergency calls. We literally lived at the veterinary hospital. After eight or nine months of being constantly on call, we protested, and the small-animal department finally included a third emergency slot, which the other faculty shared.

By the end of the year, I was tired of hassles and institutions, and I wanted to go back to California and find a nice veterinary practice. I joined a mixed practice in Carmel Valley. The owner did the large-animal ambulatory work, and I saw small animals and the large animals that came into the clinic. I treated sheep, goats, and 4-H calves but functioned primarily as a dog and cat doctor.

I wouldn't trade my year in practice for anything, because it was such good preparation for being a teacher. There is definitely a difference in clinical instructors who have been in practice and those who have not, because the economics of a private business and an institution, as well as interactions with clients, are so different.

However, I began to feel isolated in private practice and felt that I was losing capabilities that I didn't want to lose. A lot of what I was doing in practice could have been handled by a well-trained technician, while I was forgetting how to handle the really difficult cases and procedures. I finally realized that I could stay where I was and do little bits of lots of things, or I could narrow my focus and concentrate on knowing more about less. I decided to learn more about less.

I thought about what I wanted to know more about. I narrowed my fields of interest to radiology and clinical pathology. While I was at Oklahoma State, Dr. Jeffie Roszel had really piqued my interest in clinical pathology. She was very impressive in the way she showed students how to apply clinical pathology results when making a decision about care and treatment of a sick animal. I also knew that clinical pathology work required long hours at the microscope, something that tended to make me nauseated. Then one day when I was sitting at home commiserating about several of my cases that seemed to be going down the tubes, I received a call from Dr. Joe Morgan at the UC veterinary school at Davis. He asked if I would be interested in pursuing a radiology residency at the veterinary school. I told him that I needed to think about it and inquired about starting dates. Dr. Morgan said he would like me to start immediately. I decided to take the residency, and I gave my boss three weeks' notice. It seems like things open up for me at just the right time.

Half the funds for my residency came from the radiology department and half from the anatomy department. I assisted in gross anatomy and surgical-anatomy lab, and I worked with veterinary students, from freshmen to seniors. The experience in anatomy was very helpful for developing interpretive skills in radiology. Toward the end of the residency, I decided I would like to make use of my knowledge by opening a private consultation practice.

I thought San Diego would be a nice area to pursue the practice idea. I visited that city and talked to practitioners about services such as interpretation of radiographs and heart catheterizations that I could offer their patients. No one volunteered to make me a part of their staff, so I decided to wait until I had passed my radiology boards to pursue the specialty-practice idea.

I finished the residency program in June 1977 and passed the written part of the radiology board exam at that time. Everyone said the written portion of the test was the hardest, and the oral would be no sweat. Taking the board exam was the one time that I felt a lot of pressure about being female, and it was pressure I put on myself. I was told that everyone who finished the radiology program at Davis had passed their boards, and I was the first woman to complete the program and take the boards.

The oral exam covers six separate topics, and the applicant spends one and a half hours with the individual monitoring each topic. I got flustered and didn't do well on the thoracic section. I blew a couple of cases in contrast procedures, and it was downhill for the rest of the day. I knew I wasn't going to pass, and I didn't.

That was the first time I hadn't been able to accomplish something I had set out to do, and I felt like I couldn't face the people who had believed in me. I was the first woman from Davis, the radiology mecca, and I had failed.

I spent the next year reviewing a lot of radiographs, both as a relief veterinarian for radiologists in private practice and as a lecturer in radiology at the veterinary school. In 1978 I took the exam again, and this time I passed.

In the meantime, I accepted a job as a radiologist at the veterinary school at Iowa State University in Ames. This position offered the opportunity to perform clinical radiology and to teach, both of which I enjoy. The best part was having students come back and say, "I really got a lot out of your course. When I went into a preceptorship or into a practice, I was able to find things on the radiographs."

Each year I changed the way I taught radiology. I wanted to give students more than a superficial method of diagnosing from radiographs; I wanted to give them an understanding about why something looks like it does on a radiograph. We added a lecture format with extensive self-study and evaluation material. Radiology is one of those disciplines for which there are no shortcuts. You don't develop your skills until you look at lots of radiographs.

Radiographs occasionally reveal the unexpected. Several of my students who were studying gastrointestinal-tract radiology decided to practice contrast procedures for an extra-credit project. One of the students volunteered her dog, a healthy yellow Labrador retriever, as the guinea pig. They took a plain survey film, which is usual procedure, and discovered a needle in the dog's stomach. Then they administered effervescent pellets for negative contrast and were further surprised to find a ball outlined in the stomach. One enterprising student brought in an endoscope from clinics, and they managed to retrieve the needle, a red rubber jacks ball, and a pair of well-chewed bikini underpanties, all from this perfectly normal-appearing dog.

Clinical radiology is never dull or boring. It's a challenge to figure out a way to radiograph a small caged bird without scaring the little creature or restraining him too tightly. We often sedate these little fellows for their own protection. The big birds like the emus and ostriches present a different kind of problem.

We recently had an ostrich in the large-animal radiology room. The bird's owner thought the ostrich had a fractured humerus. We finally got our film but not without a struggle. The ostrich got away from the student who was holding him and ran through the room, ricocheting off the walls and skidding into tables. The poor bird seemed to have very thin skin, because he bruised and bled every time he hit another object. I was sure glad to see him go and was convinced, more than ever, that I wouldn't spend three hundred dollars for a pair of boots made out of ostrich skin.

Snakes can also be interesting patients. If you just coil a snake up, lay it on a cassette, and snap a picture, you rarely get a diagnostic film. I stretch the snake out and take views all along the length of it.

Radiographing a twelve-foot-long python or boa constrictor takes cooperation from the snake and the staff. Small lead numbers are placed consecutively down the length of the snake and close enough together so that at least two numbers will be visible on the cassette. A fourteen-by-seventeen-inch cassette is divided into three lengths, which enables us to get about four feet of snake on each cassette. If a lesion is detected on the radiograph, we can determine its anatomical location on the snake by the number.

Even if our patients are cooperative, working with x rays can be dangerous. I emphasize to students and practitioners that they are responsible, because of their training, for the people who work for them and don't have the training. Of greatest concern is the potential for harm to the fetus in the first trimester of pregnancy, especially in women who don't know they are pregnant.

Many studies have been done in human medicine concerning pregnant radiologists, and each radiology student is given these data. Sometimes we arrange to reschedule a pregnant student's radiology rotation. Other times, the student elects to continue in radiology using special precautions. We have the individual wear a 360-degree lead apron and two film badges, one at the neck and one under the apron at the waist, to monitor exposure. Adhering to standard safety practices, such as leaving the room when the film is exposed and using collimators to reduce scatter radiation, is helpful. The other radiologist on our staff at Iowa State, Dr. Elizabeth Riedesel, continued to work throughout two successful pregnancies. A practicing veterinarian who is cautious can do the same.

I think carelessness with x rays is less prevalent today than in the past. There is no doubt that placing your bare hands, or even gloved hands, in the primary x ray beam is dangerous business and increases the risk of certain cancers.

Radiation therapy for cancer in animals is another spin-off of oncology research for people. As we learn how each body system reacts to x rays, we can better utilize radiation, in combination with surgery or chemotherapy, to improve the longevity of animals with cancer.

Radiation therapy has not yet become feasible for general practitioners. The machines needed for this kind of treatment are different from diagnostic machines, and determining the correct dosage and procedure can be complicated. Computers are useful to figure the dose and size of field. Veterinary radiologists who specialize in cancer treatment often work with oncologists, human or veterinary, depending on the situation.

Ultrasound is one of the most important advances to come along in the veterinary imaging field. Ultrasound appears at this time to be harmless to patient and technician, and it gives a dynamic or moving image. Equipment is turning over so rapidly in human medical offices that veterinarians can now buy a reasonably priced used model, but it is still difficult to get the image and to interpret it. Many veterinarians who want to utilize ultrasound in their practices are taking continuing education courses to develop their skills in this procedure.

I enjoy the interactions with practitioners and students,

and I think I perform the university service and teaching roles well. But after I became tenured and was promoted to head of the radiology section, my administrative work load increased drastically. I do not think of myself as a good administrator, nor do I enjoy that role. I felt that I was being groomed for more administrative duties; I'm at the right age and I'm a woman. I also try to do a good job at whatever I'm assigned to do. I found myself getting on more committees and bigger committees.

In 1988 I was on the search committee for the new dean of the Iowa State University Veterinary School. The provost of the university encouraged us to find a qualified veterinarian who was a woman or a minority. We tried, but there were no individuals from racial minorities with significant administrative backgrounds, and women are just now becoming departmental chairs and gaining middle-management administrative experience. It will probably be a few years before we will see a minority or woman veterinarian as dean of a veterinary school or president of the American Veterinary Medical Association, which are upper-level administrative positions.

In 1988 I was also president of the American College of Veterinary Radiology. The number of board-certified radiologists has more than doubled since I sat for the boards in 1977, and at least half the applicants are women.

As my professional obligations and administrative duties increased, I became more frustrated. I worked until nine or ten o'clock at night. If I tried to get away to go camping or hiking, I faced mountains of work when I returned. Finally, what I was doing was not fun anymore. People were telling me that I was single and could do whatever I wanted. I decided to leave Iowa State, and I decided not to seek another full-time academic position.

Having a big unknown in my future is sometimes intimidating. I've elected to go west, closer to home and my family, and whenever I need a job, the people at the University of California call. I intend to set up housekeeping in the Davis area and will work at the University of California for a radiologist going on a six-month sabbatical leave, but that's it for firm commitments.

I have suffered from the belief that a good veterinarian devotes 99.9 percent of his or her time and activities to the profession. In the long run, I don't think this is in the best interest of the individual. It's important to have some time set aside for other things. Although veterinary medicine is a great career, it is only a career, and a life should include other things.

Whatever I decide to do professionally, I want to have time to do some of the nonveterinary things that I enjoy. The last few years, I have participated in community theater, and I'd like to do more of it. Ames offers at least four or five theater groups, including children's and women's theater.

I especially enjoy musicals that offer dancing parts. I have danced, primarily jazz, most of my life. It's one of my physical outlets, and I've taken lessons from time to time to hone my skills. When an interesting musical came along, I usually auditioned for a part. I've never had the lead; I'm happy to sing and dance in the chorus. The first production I did with the Ames community theater, which was "Kiss Me Kate," was my favorite because of the production's excellent choreographer and the rapport the members of the cast felt for each other. I really enjoyed that experience, and I want to have more experiences like that.

I think it is important to give something back to the community where you live. I was president of the Story County Society for Crippled Children and Adults for three years in the late eighties. We worked with business people in our area who made their facilities available to handicapped persons. We set up an equipment loan closet, as well as bowling and swimming programs.

I think people in the Midwest deserve a lot of credit for the way they support community and youth activities. I know many people from other areas of the country believe the old cliché that there's nothing to do in Iowa but watch the corn grow, but Iowans spend more time watching their children grow. Community involvement in children's school and sports activities is outstanding, and all children, not just the superstars, are encouraged to participate.

Neither my sister nor I have children, and I occasionally feel some guilt that my parents don't have grandchildren to spoil. My mother, who was a traditional role model, spent a tremendous amount of time on home and family. Because I was always such a single-track individual, I thought that I didn't have the energy to combine career and marriage. I am glad that young women of today don't feel like they have to choose between the two.

The increasing options for women reflect a positive societal trend. However, I don't think that everything is changing for the better. I have major concerns about the way society views responsibility. I saw it sometimes in students who expressed an attitude of "If I don't understand the material, it must be someone else's fault." The qualities of independence and self-sufficiency, which I admired growing up, don't seem to be valued quite as much today. Our society emphasizes consumerism, status, and consumption of resources. These things, it seems to me, will not build a long-term stable and healthy environment.

I'm very much goal-oriented. I want to be achieving something more than just a salary for myself. I thought for a long time that I was locked into being a frontline radiologist because of the time and effort I've spent on this aspect of veterinary medicine, but that's not true. It's okay to change my focus, and although that is somewhat scary, it is also challenging.

I might consider starting a consultation practice, trying my hand in industry if the opportunity presents, or working for a university on a short-term-contract basis. I don't believe in the rigidity of the university tenure system, and I think we'll see some alternative positions opening up in the academic world.

I have been involved with veterinary medicine for many years, and one of the best aspects of the profession is the quality of the individual members. Veterinarians are people who are conscientious about what they are doing, do a great job, and care about people and their animals. We don't very often have to make excuses for each other. If mistakes are made, they are usually made with the best intentions. Most veterinarians are compassionate and altruistic.

The potential in the profession is tremendous. A veterinarian is limited only by what he or she can visualize doing with the degree. I aspired to become a veterinarian when I was thirteen years old, and I still can't think of anything else I'd rather be. ■

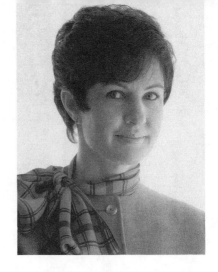

Linda M. Merry

LINDA M. MERRY is aptly named. Conversations with her are filled with merriment. "You know how we Irish are," she says before chuckling. "We laugh at wakes."

Merry's wit serves to temper the force of her driving energy, which one senses immediately upon meeting her. A flaming-A personality and an off-the-wall extrovert (her own descriptions of herself), she is a woman who will not be denied. Success for her is inevitable.

It was her do-or-die attitude that ensured that her successes would be in the field of veterinary medicine. A New Mexico State University dean sealed her fate when he said that she would never make it to veterinary school. Merry cannot resist the challenge of "You can't do that."

"Of course," she says, a grin on her face, "pioneers must expect arrows in the bustle." In the early seventies when her self-syndicated newspaper column, "The Merry Pet," was attacked by other veterinarians as being unethical, Merry refused to give it up. She continued to amuse and inform pet owners while the American Veterinary Medical Asso-ciation ethics committee investigated her and the column, not once but three times. The column was judged completely ethical and went on to win several awards.

Active in both veterinary and civic organizations, Merry has worked to promote the status of veterinary medicine and women. She is a co-owner of Alpine Animal Hospital in Pocatello, Idaho, a small city nestled in the foothills of the Rocky Mountains. Merry is also the first woman to take the helm of the American Animal Hospital Association, which has a membership of 10,500 small-animal practitioners and is the second largest organization in veterinary medicine.

Merry's accomplishments and lively leadership style have earned her numerous honors, including Idaho's Outstanding Young Woman for 1976, the Pocatello Chamber of Commerce's Athena Award, and membership in Colorado State University College of Veterinary Medicine's Distinguished Alumni.

■

I was brought up on the parable of the five talents. If God endows you with certain gifts or talents, it is imperative that you use those gifts wisely and to the betterment of God. That may translate into serving humankind or animals.

Serving animals was not always a top priority in my life. My first talent and love was ballet. From the time I was five years old, I wanted to be a ballerina, and the crucial moment in my dancing career came when I was twelve years old. My family lived at the White Sands missile base near Las Cruces, New Mexico, and my dancing teacher lived forty miles away in El Paso, Texas. My teacher pleaded with my parents to move to El Paso so she could give me intensive instruction. She promised them that at the end of three years, she would send me to New York to dance.

My father refused to consider her proposition. He told me, "Many people have bodies, but you also have a mind. If you concentrate on ballet, you will be finished by the time you are thirty years old. If you use your mind, there will never be a limit."

Regardless of his philosophy, I was crushed. I threw a big temper tantrum and generally made his life miserable. By the time I was fifteen, it was too late to be a professional dancer.

I still love to read about and attend professional ballets. However, I was forty years old before I allowed myself to dance as an amateur. Because I am so competitive, a characteristic of the flaming-A personality, I would have been heartbroken to dance and feel that I was less than the best.

Perhaps my penchant for achievement came in part from

127

being an only child and the only grandchild on both sides of my family. I also come from a line of strong-willed southerners who conquered the frontier and fought for the Confederacy in the Civil War. My grandparents all lived in Texas. Although I spent most of my adolescent years in Las Cruces, where my father worked as a mechanical engineer at White Sands missile range, I still consider Floydada, Texas, home.

My mother, with degrees in journalism and education, was a dedicated and brilliant teacher with a strong social conscience. At one time she taught a Head Start program in a black school. Another time she taught sixty first-graders, the children of migrant farm workers, who spoke only Spanish. Later, after my dad died and she remarried, she taught and lived on an Indian reservation.

My grandparents and parents are deceased now, and I feel like an orphan. I have friends who are losing their parents, and it's interesting to see the issues, many of which are left over from early childhood, that seem to surface at this time. My father, who was my mentor and emotional support, died young, at the age of forty-six, and my mother died last year.

My mother and I never shared a common philosophy of life, and we could both be considered strong personalities. The closest we ever came to a moment of truth was just prior to her death from cancer. We were having a great row, and I just stopped and said to her, "We don't agree on what's important in life, and we have different philosophies. I don't think we even like each other, but we love each other, always have, and always will." She and I stormed off in opposite directions. A few minutes later, she came back to the room where I was sitting and said, "So, do you want to play a game of Scrabble?" Scrabble, which we played ruthlessly, was our favorite family game.

My father loved animals, and I don't have a photograph of us that doesn't include a dog or cat. I think I always had a natural affinity for animals. However, I didn't consider veterinary medicine as a career until after I had graduated from high school. There was never any question that I would go to college. The questions were, Where, and what major? When I finished high school, my father asked, "What is your major going to be?"

I said, "I don't know."

My father suggested that I take a straight engineering course until I made up my mind. Well, I hate math and did not want to follow in his footsteps by studying engineering. I made up my mind fast. I would become a veterinarian.

My mother told me to forget it and consider home economics, and my grandmother, who was the real maternal figure in my life, was horrified. Grand felt that veterinary medicine was a very unladylike thing for a southern girl to do. However, my father had accepted my decision to become a veterinarian, and we marched over to New Mexico State University and met with an adviser. My father said, "Linda needs to get her schedule mapped out for preveterinary medicine."

The adviser, who was dean of the College of Humanities, said, "We've never sent a girl from New Mexico to veterinary school, and Linda's not going to make it. We just need to get her into the regular curriculum so she can get a degree when she isn't accepted."

Up to that point, veterinary medicine was probably a way out of engineering for me. But you don't tell me that I can't do something. That man's attempt to deter me from becoming a veterinarian was probably the best thing anybody ever did.

At that time, the odds were eleven to one against getting accepted into a school of veterinary medicine, and there was no pressure on the veterinary schools to accept women. New Mexico did not have a school of its own; a limited number of New Mexico students were accepted each year at veterinary schools in California, Washington, and Colorado. I was also the only female student in preveterinary medicine. Nonetheless, I was accepted by Colorado State University College of Veterinary Medicine after only two years of preprofessional courses.

Several of the men who had not been accepted were resentful of me. I remember one of my New Mexico classmates saying, "You'll never practice. You'll just get married and have kids; I would have made veterinary medicine my life's work. It's wrong, and you shouldn't be going."

I was one of three women in a class of seventy-two, and I was one of the youngest; I was nineteen when I started veterinary school. The men dropped like flies that first quarter. By the end of our freshman year, we were down to fifty-eight people. The hardest part for me was being a southern woman and competing. I was brought up to believe that you never competed with a man, at least not where he could see it. You hid your brains.

The resilient fifty-eight, including us three women, graduated in 1966. The women graduates are still practicing and have never stopped working. I worked the day my son was born and was back on the job three weeks later. My disgruntled classmate who said that the women would marry and have babies was right, but he was wrong about our failing the profession.

The three women in my class roomed together during veterinary school. I was the one who said that I would never consider marrying another veterinarian. One of my roommates married a classmate, the other married a boy in the class ahead of us, and I married a fellow in the class behind us. Never say *never*.

Jeffrey Anderson and I were married when I graduated, and I worked for the physiology department and radiology laboratory at CSU while he finished veterinary school. After his graduation, Jeff was accepted as a Purdue Fellow in the Latin America program. This program, funded by the Ford Foundation, was designed to send young professionals to Chile, Brazil, and Argentina to broaden understanding between the United States and these countries. Jeff was assigned a project to set up bovine brucellosis and tuberculosis testing programs in Argentina, but first we spent two months at Purdue University, where we received intensive training in Spanish.

Soon after we arrived in Argentina, a friend introduced me to Dr. Cora Catuogna, a woman veterinarian who had graduated from Buenos Aires University at the same time I graduated from CSU. We felt an instant rapport and decided to become partners in a small-animal practice.

Dr. Catuogna and I started the practice from scratch, and in many ways she and I complemented each other. She had better training in pharmacology because veterinarians in that country compound most of their medications, and I had superior surgical experience. We had the first clinic to offer elective surgery. We also performed orthopedic surgery, such as bone pinnings, which wasn't being done at that time; often, we used equipment borrowed from the human hospital. We dissolved the practice when I returned to the States a year and a half later. Dr. Catuogna married a fellow veterinarian and went into practice with him. She later went back to Buenos Aires University to work on a Ph.D. in pharmacology.

Back home, Jeff and I looked for the perfect town to set up practice. Jeff's area of interest was large-animal medicine, primarily equine medicine, and mine was small-animal medicine. We searched for a university city in the West that would support both large- and small-animal practitioners.

We decided on Pocatello, Idaho, the home of Idaho State University, and started the practice in a two-car garage with an attached workshop. We remodeled the clinic ourselves and lived next door. I was four and a half months pregnant when we opened the hospital.

I had always figured I was as maternal as a rattlesnake.

The idea of having a son to meet my family obligations inspired me to paint the nursery blue and select only boys' names. When my son, Worth, arrived, I proved that mind over matter works.

The night Worth was born, my grandmother came from Texas to live with us. She stayed until my son was eleven years old. I don't know of anyone I would have rather had influence him than my grandmother. Worth and I now talk about how fortunate we are to have been reared by the same wonderful person.

She was my salvation in those early years of the practice. I do not know how I could have worked the schedule that I did or accomplished what I did without my grandmother's help.

I don't buy the superwoman myth. You make a choice about what is important. I chose to go back to work when I had a child. I also gave up housekeeping and cooking. I hired someone else to do those things. Worth is in college now, and I am very pleased with our relationship. One of the reasons that we have such respect and love for each other is that I did what I wanted to do. I don't feel that I sacrificed my career for home and family.

Marriage between veterinarians puts a strain on family life because of the time commitment required. Although we tried to control competition by concentrating on different practice areas, it still existed and eventually led to the dissolution of the marriage.

When Jeff and I first worked together, I used my married name of "Anderson." In those days, a woman had to petition the courts to legally retain her maiden name. Clients called and said that they wanted Dr. Anderson, and our employees would ask, "Which one, Dr. Linda or Dr. Jeff?" I was glad to go back to my maiden name to avoid confusion and to regain it legally by divorce.

Through divorce or death of a spouse, a woman may have an opportunity to change names several times. I always counsel young women to keep their maiden names because it is so easy to lose your identity when you take your husband's name. You also lose the reputation that you have built when you change names.

I also advise young women to use "Doctor" with their names. I think that we make a mistake when we encourage our clients to call us by our first names. We give away the power of our education when we do not insist upon our title. I also think that we should show respect for our clients by calling them by their titles.

I try to encourage women to present as professional an image as possible. In corporate America, women are taught things like dress and voice modulation. We must use these tools to our advantage if we are to claim our power in the veterinary profession.

One's practice surroundings also portray a professional

image. The building that became Alpine Animal Hospital was built in 1976. The architectural goals included integrating the large- and small-animal sections while maintaining their separate functions. We drew upon our knowledge of Peruvian architecture to incorporate a lot of stone, trapezoids, and arches into the design. The result was an attractive and functional hospital certified by the American Animal Hospital Association soon after completion. In February 1978 the hospital won the Veterinary Economics Hospital Design Merit Award.

The staff at Alpine includes two associate veterinarians, a graduate veterinary technician, and seven lay employees. The relief veterinarian whom AAHA hires to replace me when I'm away on AAHA business tells me that he enjoys working at Alpine because the people like being together, work together as a team, and are conscientious about their work.

We—veterinarians and employees alike—try to stay current by attending continuing education courses. I am interested in ophthalmology and have attended several courses and wet labs devoted to this discipline. I now do the ophthalmology for the entire practice.

I knew when I became a veterinarian that I wasn't going to get rich. The internal payoff of practice for me is knowing that I've done a good job serving both animal and owner. One of my talents is working with people. I even enjoy the challenge of using my people skills on the difficult client. I have also found that I'm not going to please everybody, and I really don't care. Liberation is the realization that you don't have to care.

I have never found practice to be boring. Even if everything goes well with clients and patients, other events can make or break one's day. I recently had an awful morning that nearly made me a chocolate addict. As I walked through the hospital door at 8 A.M., my secretary handed me a notice from the Internal Revenue Service that the hospital was being audited. My soon-to-be ex-husband was waiting in the office, and we had a wonderful discussion about what he thought I should and shouldn't say in divorce court. Then the mailperson delivered a letter informing me that a job that I had been interested in had been filled. Although that wasn't a tragedy, it wasn't good news either.

I told my associate veterinarian that I thought she and I deserved a break. I suggested that we go down to the mall, buy ten of every kind of chocolate, and sit down in the middle of the mall and cry and laugh and eat chocolate until we either felt better or got sick, whichever came first. But then, practice being what it is, people kept coming in with pets, and we never got a chance to pacify our chocolate compulsions.

I have been in practice more than two decades, and I believe that a significant number of clients, especially women, have changed in the way they relate to authority figures, including veterinarians. This change, which happened at the time of the Vietnam War, is particularly evident in my generation, which fell just between the baby boomers and the old school. We either became society-oriented or became individually oriented.

People who are society-oriented are motivated by external values, and those of us who are individually oriented are motivated by internal values. Women, who used to look up to the doctor as an unquestionable authority figure, began to speak up and question decisions about their animals' care. You must earn the trust of this type of client because such clients don't give it blindly. They want to have everything explained to them, and they want to make the decisions. Because I am a person who is internally motivated, I understand and respect this type of individual, and my practice philosophy probably attracts more of these clients. Those people of the old school who seek a doctor who dictates to them will leave my practice and find a veterinarian who will give them what they want.

I like to communicate. When I found myself answering the same questions over and over in practice, I decided to address these common concerns in a newspaper column titled "The Merry Pet." The column, which was eventually picked up by nine major newspapers in seven western states, was like me: funny. The local newspaper didn't know whether to enter "The Merry Pet" in the humorous columns or the medical columns category in contests. Eventually it was first in the Idaho Press Club's syndicated columns category in 1975.

There was a need for the kind of information I dispensed in "The Merry Pet." However, in those days the American Veterinary Medical Association (AVMA) had a ban on writing for the public. I was sent before the AVMA on ethics violations three times during the seven years that I wrote the column. In each instance, the AVMA decided that the column was entirely ethical. Today many columns of this sort are in print across the United States and are considered good public relations for the profession.

I helped develop and present the public relations seminar sponsored jointly by AAHA and Gaines at our national convention, and the AAHA-Gaines public service announcements for television.

My taped radio interviews on the subject of women in veterinary medicine were aired to 266,700 listeners in the United States and Canada in 1987. I also appeared on educational television to discuss veterinary medicine in Spanish—well, maybe pidgin Spanish. People loved it. Even those who couldn't speak Spanish were intrigued at seeing me sweating it out and tongue-tied for once in my life.

I have an opportunity to communicate with both the general public and members of my profession through my involvement with AAHA. The major concern of most practitioners is economics. We are a profession struggling with a situation of making lower than professional wages. Every concern grows out of that.

The work-force issue—the worry over increasing numbers of veterinarians who must be employed—is economic. The ethics issue is economic. Our ethics problems don't involve our medical ability. We are beautifully trained. What we lack is the time, which equates to money, to continue our education. The stress issue is economic. If veterinarians made more money, they could afford to hire relief help and take more time for rest and recuperation.

More women than men are now applying to veterinary school, and the theory is being espoused that veterinary medicine is becoming a woman's profession because of low salaries. Every profession that has been feminized has lost economic buying power. It becomes a self-perpetuating downward cycle. When someone is paid less because they are female, males are less attracted also. There are more females, they are paid less, and the cycle continues.

I believe that this is primarily a female problem. We have been taught from the cradle to undervalue ourselves. We do not demand our worth. If we demand our worth from our employers, then we'll get our worth. I'm talking about the real employer—the animal owner.

Women are born to please. If you displease the guy who hires you, that is terrible. I understand it because I fight it all the time. It's a personal problem, but multiply that by 60 percent of the profession and it becomes a much larger problem.

Veterinarians are some of the most wonderful people on the earth. We have within our profession some of the greatest minds and some of the most devoted and altruistic people anywhere. However, if we are going to improve our economic power, we are going to have to believe within ourselves that we are worth it.

I think we are going to see changes in both veterinary education and veterinary licensure in the next decade. I would like to see specialty education and specialty or limited licensure accepted throughout the United States. I knew from the beginning that I was not interested in large-animal medicine, and I feel that the public would have been better served if I had concentrated my studies in small-animal medicine. If you do that in education, you must do that with licensing.

I would also like to see the acceptance of reciprocity for practitioners who wish to move to another region of the country. I never obtained a Texas license. Now twenty-plus years later, I would have to go back to school and study large-animal medicine, which I would never use again, in order to pass that test and live and practice in Texas.

I believe I should be granted a Texas license based on my proven ability in small-animal medicine in the state in which I now live and practice. Idaho cats are no different from Texas cats. An alternate idea would be to test individuals in the area of their specialty, which in my case would be small-animal medicine.

I believe in organizational veterinary medicine. I started as an affiliate member of AAHA in 1968 and became a hospital member director in 1974. By this time, I had been vice president of the Pocatello Chamber of Commerce and president of the Federation of Business and Professional Women. I had a very good organization background, but I was astounded when I sat on my first AAHA committee. These people were professionals and conducted a beautifully planned meeting that was comprehensive and complete. I felt like I was flying with eagles.

In December 1986, I represented AAHA at the World Small Animal Veterinary Association Congress in Paris. I have an interest in international relations, and this trip confirmed my view that veterinarians worldwide are more related in our concerns than we are different. In some countries, veterinarians have more prestige and better standards of living than in others, but we are basically the same.

I moved up through the ranks of AAHA, from area director to regional director to vice president and assumed the presidency in April 1989. The American Animal Hospital Association's mission is threefold—to offer programs that will enhance the ability of small-animal practitioners to offer quality medicine, to encourage practice facilities dedicated to excellence, and to serve the public's need for small-animal veterinary services. My year as president will not change the mission or direction of the organization, nor should it. I hope to be an asset to the association and to my sex.

It has been a busy but wonderful year. I have represented AAHA at regional and national veterinary meetings and several state meetings, being gone as long as four and five weeks at a time.

Organizational veterinary medicine is an area where women have been underrepresented. If women want to control their destiny and not just be pawns in it, they should take an interest in local, state, and national veterinary organizations. As a group, we can do great things. Organizations are set up to do things for you that you cannot do for yourself as an individual.

There is a lack of female leaders in organized veterinary medicine disproportionate to the number of women now in the profession. Approximately 20 percent of the nearly 46,000 members of the profession are women, and the percentage is increasing rapidly, as women account for nearly 60 percent of veterinary school enrollment. Within the American Veterinary Medical Association, only 3 female D.V.M.'s serve on committees and councils, and only 5 serve in the house of delegates out of a field of 128. Only 12 women serve on the boards of state and allied associations.

An article in *Executive Woman* magazine that I found enlightening explains what sidetracks women. If women see the game, in this case organized veterinary medicine, as dirty, they don't participate. By reacting in this manner, they automatically put themselves out of the game, and instead of being above it, they are really beneath it.

The American Animal Hospital Association is looking for women because the number of female veterinarians is increasing, especially in small-animal practice. Women who want to have a part in shaping the profession are going to have to take the time to become involved in professional organizations. We are extremely busy people, and it will have to be important enough to devote time that could be spent with the practice, the family, or an outside interest.

It takes a minimum of ten years in the trenches before an individual is ready to assume a leadership role. Leaders are made, not born. Leaders in organizations must also learn to work in teams, which is an ongoing challenge for those of us used to working as individuals. You work for the opportunity to be given more work. However, if you want to have a say, you have to play the game. The alternative is for women in twenty years to represent the majority of the profession but have no say within the profession or with the government, the press, or the public.

I don't feel that the answer is a separate association for

women. Our profession is too small to segregate by sex. I also believe that males and females are the perfect complement. We can each bring different qualities to the profession. I very much like men. I like to work with them, and I feel that it is best to have a mixture, and the more even the numbers, the better.

I have good friends of both genders, but I must give credit to four close women friends who have served as a support group for me and for each other. We are all extremely busy professional women and have to schedule time to get together. However, the support that we give each other, both personally and professionally, is invaluable.

I also give myself permission to relax and let my mind range and roam. This is important for flaming-A personalities because we are so goal- and achievement-oriented. I read voraciously, and I take time to be alone. My most creative time is from 9 to 12 P.M., which is usually time I can have to myself to read and think. Unfortunately, I sacrifice sleep, because I must get up and function the next morning at a relatively early hour.

My idea of heaven is a summer nap with a light breeze blowing through the window and a cat curled up beside me while I sleep. My cat is a real stress reliever. We have several outside and clinic cats, but I have only one personal cat at present. She is an Abyssinian, and her name is Jihan. She is named after Anwar Sadat's wife, whom I greatly admire for what she did for women.

I will soon have more freedom than I have ever had in my life. I, like so many other women, went from being someone's daughter to being someone's wife. For the first time, I will be just me, and it's like being eighteen years old again and deciding what I want to do with the rest of my life.

I am not telling myself what I have to do. When I decided to become a veterinarian, I approached that goal single-mindedly and obtained the degree in six years. I have had no time for other things, such as history and psychology, which really interest me. Because I have successfully done what I set out to do and have given over twenty-five years of my life to serving the public as a veterinarian, I think it might be okay to do something that I want for me.

I have several short stories I would like to write, but I need training. I have also contemplated pursuing a master's degree in communications. Our profession needs people who are trained in public relations. It would be fun to be a small cog in the big wheel of a huge ad campaign.

I love to travel. I have a tremendous interest in international affairs and world veterinary medicine. I would like to live in Europe long enough to get to know the people.

Once I began to give myself the freedom to think of all the things that would be fun and interesting, I thought back and knew that I could have been a ballerina and a veterinarian too. I could have danced until the age thirty and used up my body and still had time to go back to school to do anything I wanted with my brain. But we didn't allow ourselves the freedom to think that way in those days.

Just because you are a success at something doesn't mean that you have to continue doing it. I still adhere to the idea of the five talents. There might be another talent I haven't used. ∎

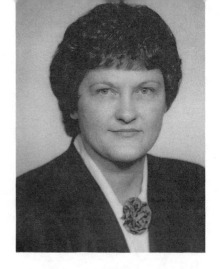

Janice M. Miller

JANICE M. MILLER, a research leader for the Agricultural Research Service of the U.S. Department of Agriculture (USDA), is an international authority on viral diseases of cattle. In 1988 Miller received two of the most prestigious awards given by the USDA: the Agricultural Research Service Distinguished Scientist of the Year Award and the USDA Distinguished Service Award.

Miller, who describes herself as a loner and a good student, knew at an early age that she wanted to solve the mysteries of animal disease by becoming a research veterinarian. After graduating magna cum laude from Kansas State University, she obtained a Ph.D. in veterinary sciences at the University of Wisconsin—Madison.

Miller is perhaps best known for discovering the virus that causes bovine leukemia and developing the test for its detection. Her picture and commentary about her findings were featured on the cover of the medical journal *Cancer Research*. Miller has authored more than one hundred research publications and presented her findings at worldwide scientific conferences. In 1977 she was voted Outstanding Woman Veterinarian of the Year by the Association for Women Veterinarians.

Miller, the fifth child in a family of six children, grew up in a small farming community in central Kansas. A quiet, gracious woman in her early fifties, she still lives by the values she learned as a youngster: work, family, and church. She is married, has two children, and lives with her family in Ames, Iowa.

■

I grew up and graduated from high school in Mentor, Kansas, a town of seventy people. My mother was a homemaker, and my father a rural mail carrier. I am the fifth child and the first of what my parents considered their second family. I was a loner and had few playmates because my siblings, except for my younger brother, who didn't come along until five years after me, were all grown and gone from home.

I developed a real love for the animals that we owned. We had dogs, cats, a pony, a cow, pigs, and chickens. The farm animals were used for milk and food, and I remember being a reluctant assistant when it came time to dress the chickens. I had expressed an early interest in becoming a veterinarian, and my mother told me that I should be able to dress chickens if I was going to be an animal doctor.

My parents' education stopped at the eighth grade, and my younger brother and I were the only children in the family to finish college. No one ever tried to discourage me from becoming a veterinarian. Some people in the community may have thought veterinary medicine was an inappropriate career for a woman, but they never mentioned it. Actually, I think they were proud of me.

I knew that I wanted to be a veterinarian because I liked working with animals, with the exception of the family chickens. During high school I became interested in science and decided that I would like to do animal disease research and find out why animals develop various illnesses and what could be done about it. I think one of the reasons I've always been drawn to research is that I like

141

mysteries. I like finding the answers to questions. There was no such thing as career counseling in those days, and it wasn't until I applied to veterinary school that I found that most people who became veterinarians did so to become practitioners, not researchers.

There were thirteen in my high school graduating class, and only one or two of us went to college. In the 1950s there was not such an emphasis on higher education.

I attended Kansas State University in Manhattan, Kansas. I knew that I had to have good grades to compete for veterinary school, but that didn't bother me, because I had always been a good student. I had an A average in my preveterinary courses, and I graduated at the top of my veterinary school class. It never occurred to me that my career wouldn't go the way I wanted, and I was never unsure of what I wanted.

I wrote down on my veterinary school application that I planned to do research when I finished professional school. I remember that Dr. Edwin Frick, who had a reputation of being tough on the women applicants, asked, "What do you think a researcher does?" I replied that I visualized a researcher going back to a lab, sitting down by herself, looking through a microscope, and finding out things. And that's the way it has turned out.

I started veterinary school with sixty-eight male classmates and one female classmate. I was never aware of any discrimination against women at Kansas State, although Vera, my classmate from Iowa, attended KSU because the veterinary school at Iowa State University did not accept women at that time. I had a lot of fun and good rapport with my classmates. I felt like I had a bunch of big brothers, and the feeling of family was one of the things that I enjoyed about veterinary school.

I also met my husband, Lyle, at KSU. We started veterinary school together that first summer, but Lyle had hurt his hand in a farming accident and dropped out to have surgery. He stayed at home for a year and started over in the class behind me. We didn't really know each other until I was a senior. Each senior was assigned a junior student for clinical rotations, and Lyle was my junior. We were teased unmercifully by our classmates when we started dating.

Lyle and I decided to marry just before I graduated. I stayed at Kansas State and obtained a master of science degree in veterinary pathology while Lyle completed veterinary school.

Pathology was an area I enjoyed. I had worked in the pathology department during veterinary school. That job consisted of typing a bibliography for one of the professors for seventy-five cents an hour. I then progressed to a research project on reticuloendotheliosis in chickens. I managed to get back to the chickens, but this time I liked it.

Two weeks after I finished my thesis defense for the master of science degree, our son, Donald, was born. Soon after, Lyle graduated from veterinary school and entered the Army Veterinary Corps. After Lyle completed his basic military courses, the three of us moved to Boston, where Lyle was assigned for one and a half years.

I wasn't in Boston long when I heard that Dr. Paul Newberne, a veterinary pathologist in the nutrition department at the Massachusetts Institute of Technology, was going to hire a veterinarian for a research project in canine distemper. I applied for the job and got it. I worked with Dr. Newberne on his project and accompanied his four graduate students to Angell Memorial Hospital for pathology seminars.

I enjoyed working with canine distemper, but I knew that I needed a Ph.D. to do research in viral-induced tumors of animals, which was really my field of interest. Dr. Newberne suggested that I contact Dr. Carl Olson at the University of Wisconsin in Madison. Dr. Olson had just obtained a grant for a project in bovine leukemia. I wrote to him about taking me as a graduate student when my husband finished his tour of duty with the army.

I don't think Dr. Olson had worked with a woman before, but he must have liked my credentials, because he offered me the chance to do my Ph.D. studies with him. I often get the feeling that some women believe that men gave them a raw deal in their careers. The people who gave me opportunities to prove myself were all men, and they took chances by accepting me. Women veterinarians were scarce then, and if I had failed, there would have been those who said to Dr. Olson and the others, "You should have known better than to take a woman with a husband and children because she'll never stick with it."

The move to the University of Wisconsin turned out well for both Lyle and me. Lyle's interest was large-animal medicine, and he had planned to look for a large-animal practice around Madison. However, when we arrived in town, Dr. Olson offered him the opportunity to obtain a master of science degree in pathology while working on the clinical part of the leukemia project. Lyle thought it was a good idea, and by the time he finished the M.S., he was so interested in pathology that he wanted to work on a Ph.D. in the field.

Lyle became the better pathologist of the two of us, because my interest was in pure research. My Ph.D. is in veterinary science, which is a research-oriented degree. I studied the effects that viruses have on disease, particularly cattle leukemia.

In 1910 the first evidence was produced that leukemia in chickens is caused by a virus. Much later, the virus that causes leukemia in mice was found. Then, in the early 1960s, the cat leukemia virus was discovered. We went to Wisconsin in 1965, and the idea behind Dr. Olson's research was to look for a virus causing leukemia in cattle.

The epidemiology seemed to prove that bovine leukemia was transmissible and was probably caused by a virus. I used the electron microscope to search for the viral particles. At first, we thought it would be easy. Most of the viruses causing leukemia in other species are readily seen by examining tumor cells in sectioned tissues or in blood under the electron microscope. I was excited about the project, but after a year of looking through the microscope and not finding anything, I thought that I was either inept or the virus wasn't there. I could have searched another twenty years and never found it, because the bovine leukemia virus is different from those viruses that had been identified at that time as causing leukemia in other species.

The bovine leukemia virus is held in the DNA of the cell. It was only when we took the tumor cells out of the blood and grew them in tissue culture that the virus was detectable. I found the bovine leukemia virus in 1969.

My discovery made it easier for researchers in the mid-1970s to find the human leukemia virus, which causes a relatively rare form of lymphoid leukemia in people. Dr. R. C. Gallo, who also discovered the HIV virus, which causes human AIDS, could not find the human leukemia virus until he took the tumor cells out of blood and grew them in tissue culture. Dr. Gallo says that viruses in all species are different, and he picks and chooses from animal research those findings that best fit his research in human diseases.

Soon after I discovered the bovine leukemia virus, Dr. Olson suggested that we develop an immunological test for its detection. An immunological test would enable us to screen cattle serum for antibodies, and we would not have to go through the time-consuming procedure of taking tumor cells and growing them in tissue culture and then looking through the electron microscope. I told Dr. Olson his idea was wrong because everyone knew that animals don't mount an immunological response to leukemia viruses. Well, that's true for the chicken and mouse, but it wasn't true for the cow. He was right. It amuses me that I am recognized for a test that I told Dr. Olson would never work.

Dr. Olson also had the idea to inoculate sheep with the cattle leukemia virus. I said, "Dr. Olson, everyone knows these viruses don't cross over into other species." We found that the cattle virus will infect sheep and will, in fact, produce tumors more often in sheep than in cattle. Because it is so difficult and takes so long for the virus to produce tumors in cattle, it was very helpful in determining that we had the right virus to be able to infect sheep with it. Dr. Olson was correct again.

I try to remember these things when I'm talking to someone about research ideas. I don't want to squelch their theories based on any type of logic, because too often logic plays tricks on you. I've had to learn the hard way to keep an open mind.

Dr. Olson was the best kind of mentor. He gave us ideas, but he also let us go out on our own and discover things in our own way. I try to mimic his style in that way when I work with young scientists.

I passed the board exam for the American College of Veterinary Pathologists soon after I obtained my Ph.D. from the University of Wisconsin. I was the second woman to be boarded in pathology. Lyle finished his Ph.D. in 1969 and took his boards after we moved to Ames, Iowa, in 1970. We were the first husband and wife team to be boarded in pathology.

Two months after I completed the thesis for my Ph.D., our daughter, Brenda, was born. I ran out of degrees and kids at the same time. I stayed at home a month when my son was born and three weeks with my daughter. I was ready to go back to work each time.

I had obtained a postdoctoral grant from the Leukemia Society of America, which supported my research while Lyle was finishing his Ph.D. After he graduated, we began looking for jobs. We liked Ames because it offered a lot of opportunities for veterinary pathologists. The Iowa State University veterinary school, as well as the U.S. Department of Agriculture's National Animal Disease Center and National Veterinary Services Laboratory, are located in Ames. Lyle got a job with the National Veterinary Services Laboratory, and I was able to transfer my grant from the Leukemia Society to the National Animal Disease Center (NADC), which is part of the Agricultural Research Service.

I was considered a collaborator at NADC because I worked on my own grant money. Then, just before my grant ran out, a job opened up, and Dr. Norman Cheville, the head of the pathology group at NADC, offered it to me.

I was the first woman scientist at NADC. Today there are thirteen women in the group of sixty-five scientists who work here. I have enjoyed the increase in numbers of women, both at the lab and at meetings, because I like discussing professional and social concerns with members of my own gender.

I suppose that I was under more scrutiny as a woman. For one thing, it was impossible to ignore me, because the men had to give up one of their locker rooms when I came. I've had friends at work say to me, "I remember when you came. You were the first woman, and we wondered how it would work out." I think this was a natural question. I never thought my gender was a handicap, and I was so self-centered in what I wanted to do that it never occurred to me that anyone would try to deny it to me.

Our business at the Agricultural Research Service is research. We work on diseases that are national in scope, and we conduct studies that build one on the other. When I came here, I continued to concentrate on bovine leukemia.

My work was first recognized in Europe. The European Economic Community made bovine leukemia one of its focus diseases and put a lot of money into sponsoring yearly conferences devoted to the disease. I presented my findings at many meetings during the 1970s. The blood test to detect animals infected with bovine leukemia virus, based on our work at NADC, was marketed by a private firm in 1978. The test is used extensively in Europe for control and eradication programs.

We received some criticism in this country after developing the test, because it was shocking to find that large numbers of cattle were infected. Some people said that the U.S. cattle industry would be better off if I hadn't discovered the virus or developed the test. I don't ever apologize for finding out things.

Bovine leukemia causes fewer problems in the United States than in Europe because here only a few infected individuals develop tumors and then only after they are four to eight years old. Most of our cattle are slaughtered before they ever reach that age. However, the Europeans are much more concerned because they keep animals longer and their herds are relatively small. The serological test helped preserve our export market, because the Europeans require proof that our exported cattle are free of the virus before they will accept them. That's a market of about $135 million in cattle and several million dollars more in semen and embryos.

For my research into the role that viruses play in cancer and my work in bovine leukemia, I was selected from a field of twenty-seven hundred scientists to receive the USDA's Agricultural Research Service Distinguished Scientist of the Year Award in 1988. I felt like it was an award for the laboratory, as well as for me. I received $40,000 in USDA support money for bovine viral research and a personal reward of $5,000.

The money was nice, but after taxes, I figured the sum had dwindled to approximately $3,000. I gave 10 percent to the church, and I was going to use the rest of the money for me. However, the day after I received the check, my daughter called from Manhattan, Kansas, where she is a student, and informed me that the engine had blown up in her car. I spent $2,400 on a new engine for Brenda's car, leaving me with about $600, and I don't know where that went.

The honor of being recognized was the ultimate reward because it meant that someone thought I had done my job well. The award is also a symbol of success, and my mom, who is a widow and over ninety years old, lived to see me excel in my profession. I hope she feels I didn't waste all their money going to school.

Soon after I received the Distinguished Scientist of the Year Award, I was chosen as one of seventeen people to receive the USDA Distinguished Service Award, which is the highest honor given by the Department of Agriculture. The ceremony, which was held in the departmental auditorium, a huge building just off the mall in Washington, D.C., was very impressive. The navy band played, and agricultural secretary Clayton Yeutter presented the awards. I felt like I was graduating again. I paraded across the stage, shook hands with Secretary Yeutter, and accepted the award.

Research is still wonderful to me. I come in on weekends, because I can't wait until Monday to see how some of the tests turn out. I am very individualistic, and I like working alone. For the most part, I've been able to work in that kind of a mode—one or two scientists working with one or two technicians on a project. However, it's becoming more difficult for an individual to work on his or her own, because science has become so complex, and research is so expensive to conduct now. It's not so easy to be a loner and make a contribution. The emphasis is more on team research with an interdisciplinary approach.

I have concentrated my work the last few years on infectious bovine rhinotracheitis (IBR). The IBR virus, which causes the disease, can cause infertility and embryonic death, and the modified-live-virus vaccines used to prevent the disease can cause abortions in pregnant cows. It is important to develop safer vaccines. Many people are questioning the use of animals as research models. However, the ultimate research test for the study of diseases like IBR is the animal experiment. You cannot duplicate reproductive function or the interrelationships of the endocrine organs in the test tube.

Now that I am a research leader, I am involved more with people and with meetings. I oversee a staff of seventeen people and a $1.3 million budget, and that means more time that I must spend on administration and less time that I can spend doing research. It has made me appreciate the administration and organization that makes research possible, but I hope to go back to full-time benchwork soon.

In research, you can design your own hours and can be your own boss. If I take off for fifteen minutes, I take fifteen minutes of annual leave, and that way I feel no guilt. Most of us put in more than forty hours a week, but the hours can be somewhat flexible. I think it's a nice career for a veterinarian with family obligations.

I don't encourage or discourage young people who are considering veterinary medicine as a career. The road to becoming a veterinarian is so long and hard that the individual must really have an intense desire to do it. If school isn't fun, the degree may not be worth it. I don't think it's a good idea to encourage young people beyond their capability and desire, and if they want it bad enough, they probably won't be easily discouraged.

I decided from the beginning that I liked my work, but I didn't intend to sacrifice my life for it. My family, my church, and my community—those things are important too.

I am glad that Lyle is a veterinarian and we share the same discipline. I'm so wrapped up in what I'm doing, and that's all I want to talk about. I don't think a husband in another career field would understand. Our history goes back to the same people in veterinary school. He now works at Iowa State University, and I know people there. He knows the people where I work. We go to meetings and have the same friends and acquaintances. Veterinary medicine is our family.

We have enjoyed living in Ames because it is small yet offers many of the advantages of a large city because of the university. We enjoy college sports, especially football, basketball, and wrestling. We are both active in our church. I was raised in the Methodist church, and it's a natural part of our life.

I think this has been a good place to raise children. Our

daughter is majoring in interior design at our old alma mater, Kansas State, and we like going back there for visits. Our son, Don, teaches biology in Des Moines, so he shares our interest in science. His wife, Mary, is also a teacher. We are traveling more since the children are gone, and we'd like to do more of it.

I have great empathy for the people in my section who have dual-career families, and almost all of them do. These young scientists can't give eighty to ninety hours a week to their jobs. Some of the older administrators, who devoted their lives to their jobs and had wives at home to take care of family responsibilities, probably can't deal with this as well as I do.

I see a different attitude toward work coming from the younger scientists. They are beginning to question what authority figures say is right or expected; they are taking responsibility for molding their lives and careers. They seem to be saying, "I'm willing to work, and I'm dedicated—but not to the point of giving my body and soul or the rest of my life." I see this as a positive change. It is not in society's best interest to have people devoted to their work to the exclusion of everything else.

Today's generation feels less threatened by changing jobs or careers. It's acceptable to be mobile, and a lot of people need change. I think this is a selling point of veterinary medicine. It's such a broad profession that people can change jobs and directions within the profession. I don't seem to need that change. I'm extremely satisfied with my job.

The profession has provided me with a comfortable income. My main indulgences, in terms of money, are a nice car and a new house. I think I enjoy those things because we didn't have them when I was growing up. Because my dad was a rural mail carrier, he always drove a car that was splattered with mud, and we lived in an older house.

My job means much more than money to me. The work is interesting, and I feel like I have made a contribution to society. You can't ask for more than that from a career. ∎

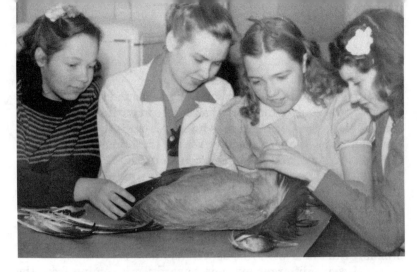

Patricia O'Connor Halloran

WHEN Patricia O'Connor took her place as veterinarian at Staten Island Zoo, New York, in 1942, the five-foot-one, twenty-six-year-old mother of two became an overnight sensation. Reporters flocked to photograph the first female zoo veterinarian in the United States and quite possibly the world. Dressed in nylons, heels, and skirt, protected only by a white lab coat, O'Connor was pictured while she pilled alligators, extracted an infected tooth from an anesthetized cougar, and hefted the coils of a twelve-foot boa constrictor. Her youthful portrait appeared everywhere, even on an ad for New Departure Safety Brakes in which O'Connor was described as "a champion" and was given a one-paragraph biography as part of the company's scrapbook of famous American outdoorsmen. O'Connor kept the spotlight on herself and Staten Island Zoo, nationally and internationally, for an unprecedented twenty-eight years.

O'Connor graduated in 1939 from Cornell Veterinary College in Ithaca,

New York, and joined 31 women in the profession nationwide. By 1964, when the number of female veterinarians had swelled to 277, O'Connor was not only their prime mentor but also one of the most famous and admired veterinarians in the United States.

She began her zoo practice in the days before textbooks or college courses on diseases of wild animals. Anesthetics were limited to capsules of pentobarbital sodium hidden in food, and ether poured on a large cotton wad. Necessary information was exchanged by word of mouth among the seven or eight full-time U.S. zoo veterinarians and their animal curators.

Using methods of disease prevention and control learned in veterinary college and deducing treatments for wild animals from their domestic counterparts, O'Connor kept detailed records of her own observations. She carefully autopsied every zoo animal that died to search for the cause of death. She also started a card file listing any helpful references she could find on wild-animal disease, and the project soon grew beyond just personal interest. O'Connor received the first grant given by the National Institutes of Health for a bibliography. The grant inspired her ten-year task of compiling references on wild-animal disease from more than eight thousand articles found in more than nine hundred publications. In 1955 the American Veterinary Medical Association published her book, *A Bibliography of References to Diseases in Wild Mammals and Birds.*

In addition to guarding the health of 780 animals, O'Connor taught science and advanced biology to elementary and high school students. Classrooms, a laboratory, and a large auditorium established Staten Island Zoo as a pioneer in public education. O'Connor remembers, with great pleasure, that many of her students followed careers in medicine and veterinary medicine.

A revered authority on wild animals, O'Connor traveled around the world visiting more than fifty countries and one hundred zoos. She likes to recall a zoo in India where chamber music was played and tea and cakes were served to the visitors. Speaking at several American Veterinary Medical Association conventions, she often attracted the lion's share of the press with her zoo and wildlife topics. In 1964 O'Connor was given the honor of presenting a paper entitled "Diseases of Captive Wild Animals" at the International Veterinary Congress in Hannover, Germany. Today she is a life member of the American Association of Zoo Veterinarians and a fellow in the New York Academy of Science. A gifted communicator not only

as a teacher and a scientific speaker, O'Connor wrote more than fifty animal portraits for the Staten Island Zoo bulletins, two chapters for the first edition of the *Merck Veterinary Manual,* and a chapter on diseases of snakes in the 1966 *Current Veterinary Therapy.*

To assuage her fierce desire to learn, O'Connor completed postgraduate courses given by Walter Reed Army Medical Center, Harvard Medical School, the Centers for Disease Control in Atlanta, Lincoln Park Zoo in Chicago, and the Animal Medical Center in New York City. During fifty years of practice she attended thirty American Veterinary Medical Association conventions and three International Veterinary Congresses. Chosen Outstanding Woman Veterinarian of the Year in 1956 by the Association for Women Veterinarians, she was named Woman of the Year a few years later by the Staten Island Soroptimist Club and the College of Staten Island.

At age seventy-five in 1990, O'Connor still practices small-animal medicine at Halloran Animal Hospital. She inherited the hospital from her husband, whose father had built it next to his own father's blacksmith shop. The antique portrait of her father-in-law, who once boarded a circus elephant, peers at clients in the waiting room. Still slender, in heels and a silk dress imprinted with blocks of vivid color, O'Connor steps lively, and her round, animated face, softened by auburn hair, is ageless.

■

I attended my fiftieth class reunion in Ithaca, New York, this year [1989], and everyone was bragging about what little money they made when they first graduated. One fellow got up and said his first office-call charge was two dollars, and after fifty years, he still hadn't collected it. Another classmate, who drove the ambulance for the county hospital in Ithaca, collected fifty cents a night. Now most of my classmates are retired, except for two who are teaching in medical schools. Out of my class of forty, with three women, eleven have died, including my husband.

My husband, John Halloran, wanted me to use my maiden name, O'Connor, to prevent client confusion. John had a wonderful sense of humor. When anybody brought a gerbil or parakeet to his hospital and he was too busy to bother, he would tell the client that Dr. O'Connor, at the zoo, was a specialist in gerbils or parakeets. He never let on that we were married and thought that was a huge joke.

I was born in New York City, but my father died when I was three months old. Mother returned to her family in Buffalo, and I grew up there. My grandmother kept cows, only three at a time, and across the road from her house were fields where we picked wild strawberries. I had many dogs and cats and liked to pretend they were patients in my animal hospital. Coaxed with candy pills, they had to allow their legs to be bandaged. I also hung around an animal hospital in Buffalo and thought it was wonderful when they let me clean the cages or walk the dogs. My mother assumed that my animal phase would pass. Mother went only through the tenth grade, but as I get older, I think she was really smart.

My stepfather graduated from a Catholic college and worked in real estate. As a bigwig in Buffalo's chamber of commerce, he was chairman of the greeters' committee. Mother and I often met famous people like Cardinal Pacelli and Babe Ruth. When the chamber opened the Peace Bridge from Buffalo to Canada over the Niagara River, the Prince of Wales came for the ceremony. Our maid was so excited that she bought a new dress to meet the prince, but even Mother and I didn't get to sit on the dais.

I started writing to Cornell Veterinary College when I was in high school so they would know I was serious. They didn't seem to have strong opinions either way about women. By the time I graduated from high school, the Depression had settled, and I didn't think I could afford college. I worked in a department store for one year. Then a wealthy aunt died and left me sixteen thousand dollars.

I went to the University of Alabama for my preveterinary

work, which in 1934 was only one year. It was easy to get on the dean's list at Alabama, so Cornell Veterinary College accepted me. Because the university charter at Cornell would not allow a majority of one religion on its board of trustees, my relatives scolded Mother for allowing me to go to the so-called "godless school on the hill."

Florence Kimball was the first woman to graduate from Cornell in 1910. I didn't know her, but I knew Elinor McGrath, who graduated in 1910 from Chicago Veterinary College. [Kimball and McGrath were the second and third female veterinarians to graduate in the United States.] Dr. McGrath was a little bitty thing, but she was fun. She told us at a meeting of the Association for Women Veterinarians that her male classmates complained so much about having a woman in class that she went to the dean and volunteered to leave. "No," he told her. "You'll make a better veterinarian than any of them."

Many of my classes were at the agriculture school. We had to judge livestock and know all the grains and hays and how to calculate nutritious diets. All the emphasis was on food animals. We learned anatomy on the horse. There was also a course in horseshoeing. Women could take the lecture but were not allowed in the lab where students actually fitted shoes on horses. I received an A for that lab and never once saw a horse shod.

While a student, I worked every summer for a veterinarian in Brockport, New York, twenty miles from Rochester. My pay was room and board, and it was the best thing that ever happened to me. In his animal hospital the veterinarian had a room with twenty cages, and I scrubbed every cage every day. He filled them with dogs to be boarded and a few small-animal patients, but he mostly treated farm animals. I rode the countryside with that veterinarian, and he made me talk to the farmers. If I said a horse had tetanus, he'd tell me, "That farmer doesn't know what you mean. Say the horse has lockjaw." At veterinary school, girls were not permitted to go on ambulatory, but my work in the Brockport practice gave me more ambulatory experience than any student in my class. The last time I drove back to Brockport, there was a big shopping mall on the spot where once I had looked out the kitchen window at dairy cattle grazing in a green pasture. I could have cried.

Oddly enough, Cornell Veterinary College saw nothing wrong with women doing rectal exams on cattle, so I did a lot of those. [The manure is cleaned from a cow's rectum and the examiner reaches his or her entire arm, protected by a lubricated sleeve into the rectum until the uterus and other structures in the pelvic cavity can be felt through the rectal wall.] I remember going to a fancy ball with a beau from the agriculture school. My date took me someplace to have a drink before the dance, and there I recognized one of my classmates. I was dressed in a long, lacy gown with white kid gloves up to my elbow. My classmate came over and whispered, "All I can think of is you doing a rectal on that cow this morning."

One time my classmates chose me to clean the smegma [a thick, smelly glandular secretion] out of the sheath on a stallion's penis. They were hoping for a big laugh if I refused, but I surprised them and did it. A lot of things stunk in veterinary medicine. Even the medications we used for skin problems had a terrible odor.

My first job after graduation was in Charleston, West Virginia, working for a small-animal practitioner who was also chief veterinarian for the health department. I learned a great deal about public health. My boss was responsible for men who inspected kitchens in all the restaurants. We received many health department calls at the animal hospital from people who were usually angry with my boss.

John Halloran was my classmate. He was older because he had graduated from college and taught before he entered veterinary school. We graduated in June of 1939 and were married in September of 1940. John worked for his father, who had built a horse hospital in 1902 on Staten Island. My father-in-law used to make his calls in a horse and buggy, and I've kept the silhouette of a horse and buggy on my stationery for my logo.

When I first came to Staten Island, there were three hundred head of dairy cattle here, and my husband did all the testing for tuberculosis and brucellosis. There were a few goats and pigs to vaccinate, and across from the house where I now live, sheep used to graze. My husband worked seven days a week. He loved the horse work. There were several riding academies and some horses owned by individuals.

During my first year of marriage, I was so gung ho that I spent every day at the animal hospital. We'd split the surgery, and then I'd do house calls. I put all my earnings in the hospital cash box. My father-in-law paid my husband only two hundred dollars a month, and out of that we paid rent for our apartment. I worked up until the day my son, John Halloran III, was born. He says that's why he is always so tired.

While I was in the hospital, my mother came to my home to help. She wanted to rest alone in my apartment after her trip, but the relatives insisted she see the sights. With all the attention, she was so uncomfortable that I signed myself out of the hospital early to be with her. In those days they wanted new mothers to stay in the hospital ten days. Now they kick you out in three. I told the obstetrician, "I can't see making such a fuss over having a baby. The Indians had their babies without any doctors." I used to brag at veterinary meetings that I worked up until the day each of my three children was born. But the men always assured me their wives were just as rugged.

My mother left after two weeks, and I returned to work part-time. On my day off, I had just put a cake in the oven when my husband called and said he needed me right away to hold a parrot for minor surgery. I wrapped my son in a blanket and left him with my mother-in-law, who lived near the hospital. I helped my husband, drove back, picked up my son, and got home just in time to take the cake out of the oven. Other times, I took the baby with me, strapped him into his infant seat, and set him in one of the animal cages.

I never was paid for my work at the animal hospital. I figured my father-in-law owed me two thousand dollars just for mileage on my car at the current rate then of five to six cents per mile. I was delighted when the Staten Island Zoo called because I wanted an excuse to leave practice. I started to think, What would my husband do if his wife wasn't a veterinarian?

In truth my father-in-law was always good to me. As he aged, he developed a special distaste for stoplights. Because he lived on the island before stoplights, he felt no obligation to stop. Whenever I could, I'd drive him on his calls, or we'd go to horse sales together.

My father-in-law was well known for his horse knowledge. He bought horses for the police department, and we boarded five police horses in the old blacksmith shop behind the hospital. One time Snug Harbor, a retirement home for old sailors, asked my father-in-law to find them a team of draft horses. I drove him to Freehold, New Jersey, from one sales barn to another, and nothing he saw suited him. We planned to return in a week when they received new horses. In the meantime, the so-called governor of Snug Harbor fancied himself a horseman and picked out a team we had turned down. My father-in-law was still paid a commission, but in two weeks the team was lame.

When the zoo interviewed me, I was pregnant with my second child. She was born in September, fourteen months after John, and we named her Patricia O'Connor Halloran. I started work at the zoo in October 1942, when I was twenty-six years old. I replaced my husband's cousin. When he left, the zoo knew they couldn't find a man during the war, so they called me. Before I took the job, I called my friend Dr. Leonard Goss [director of the Cleveland Zoo and formerly veterinarian of the Bronx Zoo], who told me the zoo people couldn't expect to find anybody with previous zoo experience. As it turned out, they were delighted to get anybody. I figured I'd work until the war was over, but I stayed twenty-eight years. Now I collect a pension from the zoo, because it was a city job. The zoological society ran the zoo, but the city paid the bills. When the zoo first opened in 1936, the governing board applied for a teacher, but the city fathers said they'd rather pay for a veterinarian.

Staten Island had one of the first educational zoos. We had classrooms and a big auditorium. Nature study class was every afternoon for elementary-age children. The scientific staff—the director, the curator, and I—took turns giving lectures. My favorite class was high school biology. Once a week four students from each high school, selected by the head of their biology department, showed up full of enthusiasm for my noncredit course. I introduced them to the microscope and the microtome and used skeletons, charts, and live animals to teach comparative anatomy. At the end of class, I began autopsies for those who wanted to watch. All the teens stayed and loved it. One boy said to me after an autopsy, "That was cool!" I didn't even know what *cool* meant.

Many of my former students became veterinarians or medical doctors. One is now on the faculty at Cornell. It's fun to hear what becomes of them. One was part of the team of doctors who delivered Luci Baines Johnson's baby, and another works for the Pentagon. I know because a government agent visited me to check on him. During my years with the zoo, I gave lectures about animal care to people of all ages. I remember special programs for servicemen and foreign women who were taking English classes in Manhattan. I always brought live animals, especially snakes so children and adults could handle them and learn not to be afraid.

Zoos began as private animal collections owned by wealthy people. The zoo in Copenhagen is next to the palace and at one time belonged to the king. At first the public was allowed entrance only one day a week.

Staten Island Zoo, with its six hundred to eight hundred specimens, was a private estate at one time, so its space was limited. We never had an elephant, but we had all the big cats, a variety of monkeys, and one of the biggest and most complete reptile collections in the world. Our orangutans had the strength to bend their cage bars and the dexterity to loosen screws in the floor drains with their fingernails. We had the first baby chimpanzee born in New York City. I hand-raised that baby. Recently a newspaper article said Central Park Zoo had the first chimp baby. I should have called the paper.

When I was traveling in Malay, north of Singapore, my veterinary group took a tour of a snake farm. The local reptile men boasted about their unusual collection, but most of the snakes I had seen and handled at Staten Island.

Zoos are the most usable form of recreation. They appeal to all age groups in all weather, unlike a golf course or even a swimming pool. The Staten Island Zoo was open every day, and I worked many Christmases. Now it closes on holidays. I worked five days a week, nine to five, but I was always on call and often gave evening lectures.

I had full charge of the animal collection. I planned the animals' diets, supervised their feeding, treated the sick, and even did surgery. I autopsied every animal that died and was baffled when I discovered that some larger zoos didn't. There was a tremendous lack of information about the cause of wild-animal deaths. Nutrition was very important. Many captive birds lost their brilliant color on an improper diet. While flamingos at other zoos faded, ours regained their rich salmon color when I supplemented their diet with sufficient fresh beta-carotene, a precursor of vitamin A. During World War II, military personnel had priority for many foods, and I had to find satisfactory substitutes for scarce items. Fresh bananas were not available for the monkeys, so we fed them dehydrated bananas and sweet potatoes. For the carnivores, we substituted horsemeat for beef. Many of my food problems were solved when I devised a basic, pelleted ration. We thoroughly ground and mixed essential ingredients like cereals, liver, bonemeal, fish, cheese, dried milk, and soybean meal. Cod liver oil, at the proper dose, was given daily as a supplement, and animal health improved.

In counsel with the keepers, I learned to prevent many problems. Sometimes two or three weeks would go by without a sore paw or any serious illness. The animals were my business associates, and every morning as I made rounds, I called to them by name. I'd hold the hands of the monkeys so they became accustomed to putting their arms through the bars. This made it easier to give injections when they were needed.

Anesthetics in the early days were very limited. I could hide Nembutal [pentobarbital sodium] capsules in food and wait, sometimes eight hours, until the animal was safe to approach, or place an animal in a squeeze cage with ether-saturated cotton. We'd cover the cage with heavy canvas and wait until the animal was groggy enough to handle. Once we could touch the animal, we could give sedatives by injection. For short procedures, small animals were restrained in nets and held with heavy gloves. Large animals, like wildcats, were pinned against the bars of the squeeze cage to expose an injection site.

After I took a postgraduate course in orthopedic surgery from Dr. Jacques Jenny, I repaired all uncomplicated fractures myself. My husband helped me with some patients, but if I was really stumped, I called my circle of well-informed veterinary friends. A physician on the board of zoo trustees helped me when one of the chimps and several other monkeys developed tuberculosis. After the first outbreak, we tested all incoming primates to make sure they didn't have TB, then retested them one year later. The monkeys caught TB from the public, so we placed all our monkeys behind glass. The people always thought the glass was for their own protection.

I don't recall any one animal being more difficult to treat, but some of the wild-caught birds didn't adjust well to captivity. Once we had a hyena we wanted to load into a shipping crate and send to the Bronx Zoo. He wouldn't eat the medicated meat, and it took us four days to entice him into the crate. When the capture gun became available, it was a great help. In our small cages the animal was easy to hit with the anesthetic dart.

My friend Estelle Geller, a veterinarian in charge of laboratory animals at Albert Einstein College of Medicine, came to the zoo with her technician to collect blood from a chimp. One of the doctors at the medical center wanted to transplant the chimp's liver into a human. The chimp didn't show much effect from my first sedative dose, so I gave her more. The technician drew her blood sample, but the chimp dropped into a very deep sleep. Her body temperature fell to ninety-four degrees Fahrenheit. I brought my electric blanket from home and stayed with her all night, turning her regularly. She finally woke up and lived to have three or four young. The people on the island knew all the animals by name, and they would have missed that chimp. Fortunately she wasn't needed for the liver transplant.

The zoo hospital was on the second floor, and that was

where we quarantined all new animals for thirty days. A young orangutan wouldn't walk downstairs to the exhibition cage. I was pouring a spoonful of Thorazine syrup [a tranquilizer] for him when he suddenly reached out, grabbed the almost-full bottle and drank the entire contents. That night the watchman called and said the male orang was very restless and acting strangely. At 2 A.M. I called the drug company that made Thorazine. The veterinarian told me to give the orang a little Demerol. I rushed to the zoo to dose him, and he soon returned to normal.

People often brought sick exotics to me or injured native wildlife, like raccoons and opossums. I never charged them but did what I could for the animal. Even the Bronx Zoo sent people to me. If people insisted on paying, I told them to put money in the zoo contribution box.

One woman had several pet monkeys, and for a person who kept monkeys, she was quite reasonable. I was treating her woolly monkey when she called and said the monkey died.

"Where is the body, now?" I asked.

"We buried it," she said.

About an hour later she called me back. "Why did you want to know where the monkey was?"

"I thought it would make an interesting autopsy," I told her. So she dug it up and brought it in. She dealt with an animal importer in New York, and after that she brought me all the dead monkeys from the importer.

Lisbeth Kraft, a veterinarian who worked for the New York City Health Department, wanted to set up a testing station on Staten Island to see if our mosquitoes carried eastern equine encephalomyelitis. The zoo trustees approved the testing, so Lisbeth sent a big cage, stocked first with pheasants, then quail. Technicians from New York's health department came once a month to draw blood samples from the birds. This was the only real research project we had at the zoo.

I kept records of all animal exchanges and purchases, so I knew how much every animal cost. In India I was trying to buy cobras, and the locals thought I was strange. I saw some fellow playing a pipe to entice snakes out of a basket, and I told him I wanted to buy his snakes. In his Indian dialect he kept chattering so many rupees. The price sounded like a very good deal, so I told him I'd buy all his snakes. What he really meant, I found out later, was so many rupees to take his photograph.

When I was on a trip around the world with the California

Veterinary Medical Association in 1965, the director of the Tokyo Zoo, whom I had met in the United States, insisted I tour his zoo. I'd been on the plane many hours, but my schedule in Tokyo was so full that I went immediately to his zoo. After walking the grounds for three hours, I admired the raccoon dogs, so the director gave me three pairs. Common in Japan, the raccoon dogs were a popular new attraction at Staten Island. I wanted to return the favor and tried to think of an interesting animal for the Japanese. Finally I shipped three pairs of Virginia opossums. The director sent me newspaper clippings of the elaborate Japanese ceremony, complete with a band, that celebrated the arrival of the opossums. I felt guilty that I hadn't had a ceremony for the raccoon dogs.

Every year I went to the International Zoo Veterinarians meeting in Europe. The Europeans put us to shame the way they entertain. One year I went a week early to spend time in East Berlin with veterinarians I'd met the year before. Every night we went to the home of a different veterinarian and had a party. Then we all went to Zagreb, Yugoslavia, for the zoo meeting. When the second week was over, I was too exhausted to go to Ireland as planned and stayed in Frankfurt a week to rest.

On my trip to China in 1981, I saw surgery performed on a cow while acupuncture was used for anesthesia. It was very impressive. The animal lay quietly, chewing her cud during the operation, then jumped up afterward as though nothing had happened. I bought an acupuncture set, but the U.S. customs official at the airport wanted 100 percent duty on any product made in Red China.

I objected. "That was the whole purpose of Nixon going to China," I told him.

"Are you a doctor?" he asked. Then he discussed it with his superior, and they let me go without paying duty.

At home one of my responsibilities was to lecture to customs inspectors on Staten Island regarding the recognition of birds in the parrot family. Imported parrots could carry serious disease, and the identity of psittacine birds was made difficult by their enormous range in size.

During World War II, scientists wanted to establish primate centers to provide a reliable source of healthy monkeys for testing the polio vaccine. I was one of about sixteen people invited to Washington, D.C., all expenses paid, to help establish these centers.

Animals in a zoo often achieve their full life expectancy. A herring gull can live fifty-five years in a zoo, or about 75 percent longer than in the wild. Veterinarians and physicians always wanted hearts and aortas from older zoo animals who died, for the study of atherosclerosis. One scientist collected prostate glands from old male animals, and another wanted only brains.

From the moment I began work at the zoo, I collected references on wild-animal diseases for my own satisfaction. At some point I realized the great need for an organized, up-to-date reference on articles concerning diseases in wild animals. As my file grew, I applied for a National Institutes of Health grant. Mine was the first grant issued for a bibliography. Before I started my book, I wrote to the department of natural resources in every state and explained my interest in wild animals. At that time, surprisingly, very few were interested in conservation. Most of my references were compiled in the libraries of the New York Academy of Medicine and the American Museum of Natural History. I listed all pertinent articles covering a period of 120 years (1830–1950), including those in foreign languages. After ten years of reviewing more than nine hundred publications, I hired a professional typist to prepare the final 1,410-page manuscript. The book, *A Bibliography of References to Diseases of Wild Mammals and Birds,* was published by the American Veterinary Medical Association in 1955. The demand was greater than the number of copies printed. By 1962 the book was available only as a reprint of a microfilm-Xerox. I still get letters from people who want a copy.

My younger daughter was born eighteen months after I became zoo veterinarian. I treated a cougar the day before her birth and took only a ten-day maternity leave. By then my mother lived with us, and I often say to my son, "I don't know how Grandma managed." She watched three grandchildren and cooked and cleaned while my husband and I worked. I had a man disk the vacant lot next to our house, and Grandma planted a victory garden. She was delighted with her garden plus doing all the housework.

One of our house pets was a South American parrot that I brought home to save from constant pecking by his fellow parrots. Mother entertained her friends at the beauty parlor with stories of the bird's newest sayings. As she came up from the basement one day, the bird told her, "There's somebody at the door."

"Which door?" she asked the bird. "Front or back?"

The bird slowly shifted to one leg, raised his other foot, and pointed.

All my children worked in their father's animal hospital, but none wanted to be a veterinarian. The work was too hard.

People called the house constantly, even while my husband ate dinner. I'd tell people he was at a meeting. My daughter said I told people Daddy was gone so often that they'd begin to think he was a rounder.

My husband was good friends with the director of the Animal Medical Center in New York City. Once a week at the center a noted outside speaker lectured. For that day, I worked in my husband's practice, and he would take the speaker to lunch or dinner.

My husband kept animals owned by the U.S. Public Health Service in his hospital. He was paid board and a fee when doctors used his operating room. He would have forsaken the money for the marvelous opportunity to watch human surgeons pioneer work that led to grafting blood vessels around the heart. Eventually the Public Health Service built its own facility, and my husband became its consultant. After his death, they made me consultant.

When my younger daughter was of college age, we bought a thick book describing U.S. colleges and wrote to about forty-five of them. I discovered a college in New Orleans that said, "Spend your junior year in Switzerland." There was a little asterisk beside the name. I thought Switzerland sounded nice, so I wrote to the college. Later my daughter complained, "Mother, don't you know what that asterisk means? You wrote to an all-black college. They'll think I'm a freedom rider."

She finally went to St. Mary's in South Bend, Indiana, where she met her future husband, a law student at Notre Dame. Now she has her master's degree from Notre Dame because the two colleges merged. She still lives in South Bend and has three children. The oldest just graduated from Notre Dame.

My older daughter lives in St. Louis with her family. My son, Jack, who never married, lives with me and helps me with the animal hospital.

My husband died in 1966, and I inherited Halloran Animal Hospital. For a few years I worked both the zoo and, at night, the animal hospital. At age fifty-five, I retired early from the zoo.

When I left, the zoo used my salary to hire three keepers, which they needed more than a full-time veterinarian. They also built a new zoo hospital. The hospital cost more than the original zoo. The zoo always seemed nice to me on its small budget. The grounds were landscaped and homelike, all the trees were labeled, and many people came just to relax. Now I seldom go to the zoo. Staten Island continues to expand. High-rise apartments for low-income residents have replaced a nearby island golf course.

When my husband practiced, the only veterinarians on the island were he and his father, an old veterinarian on the boulevard, and Dr. John Ward, the zoo vet in 1937 who started his own practice in an old house in 1939. Now there are ten animal hospitals and thirty veterinarians. My classmate from Scottsdale, Arizona, said in Scottsdale there was a veterinarian on every corner. That didn't mean much to me until an emergency clinic opened a block away from my hospital. My profession is going to degenerate not because there are too many women but because there are too many veterinarians.

My son, Jack, and I operate the animal hospital. Jack, as my receptionist and helper, keeps the building in repair and buys all the drugs. We don't bill, which makes less work. My hours are evenings from five to seven and twelve to three on Saturdays. Most of my clients work, so these hours suit them. When my husband died, I changed my home phone to an unlisted number. I tell people to use the young vet who opened the emergency clinic near me if they need service after hours.

I don't do bone work now. I perform routine surgeries, like spays, castrations, and dentistry. The other day I did a pyometra [removed an infected uterus], but I'd rather not do those. I refer difficult surgeries. Let the young people sweat them out.

I walk the big dogs up the stairway to the surgery room before I induce anesthesia. If the dog is heavy and my son is not around, I ask a neighbor at the garage or the grocery to help lift the dogs onto the table.

The brick walls of the animal hospital are eighteen inches thick, and except for the stone and windows that fill the space where barn doors opened for the horses, they've been standing since 1902. The cages have thick plywood floors waterproofed by a heavy marine varnish, the ceilings are high, and the old rooms spacious. I am the last heir, and I can't bear to sell.

A cute young couple came in the other day and said they'd taken their cat to three veterinarians, and it was still sick. Someone finally told them, "Take your cat to the little old lady on Broad Street. If she can't fix him, nobody can." I still feel satisfaction when an animal recovers, especially if it has been to another veterinarian. Maybe it would have gotten better by itself—who knows?—but I get the credit.

An old-time client brought me his sick Afghan hound. I felt the dog was dying but sensed the old man wasn't prepared to hear this. I gave the poor dog injections to make him feel better. On my day off, the old man took his dog to another veterinarian who ran endless laboratory tests, then sent the man and his dog to the Animal Medical Center in New York. There the dog soon died. Afterwards I met my old friend in the bank and asked him how much money he spent on his dog. "Over a thousand dollars," he said.

I was mad. The other veterinarian should have known that even a thousand dollars couldn't save that fourteen-year-old Afghan from dying. Yet it's strange. Although I may suggest euthanasia, some people insist on keeping the animal alive. One woman had a cat with diabetes. I told her to take it to the Animal Medical Center, but that it would cost a lot of money to treat.

"I don't care," she said. "I'll put a mortgage on the house."

Two days later she called and asked, "Will you put the cat to sleep?"

I don't think it's proper for a professional to advertise in the yellow pages. I don't try to sell anything. I don't sell dog food or groom, bathe, or board. I don't send out vaccination notices. I tell my clients to come back, and they do if they want to. I give people pamphlets from the American Veterinary Medical Association if they want information, but I don't tell them they have to do anything.

I enjoy the people in my practice. If people come in with a chip on their shoulder, I say, "I think you'd be better off with another veterinarian." Then they do an about-face. "But I've always come here," they say. "My mother came here, and my grandmother." There are a lot of new people on the island, but I have some clients who have stayed with me for three generations.

My friend is dean at one of the colleges here and asked me to represent veterinary medicine on career day. I had a table stacked with leaflets on veterinary careers. A young minority student picked up a leaflet. "How much does a vet make in a year?" he asked.

"Well," I told him, wondering what he had in mind, "if you work full-time you could net fifty thousand dollars."

He put the pamphlet back. "I'm only interested in something that pays a hundred thousand dollars," he said.

I blame black leaders for using millionaires like Sammy Davis or famous athletes as role models for these children. When the kids can't fulfill these impossible goals, they go into drugs or crime.

Taxes are my hobby. I study legal tax avoidance, not tax

evasion. Recently I've taken courses on estate planning and real estate.

I attended the World Small Animal Veterinary Association Congress in Harrogate, England, in 1989. I traveled with retired veterinarians, and we had a private reception for James Herriot and other big wheels in the British small-animal association. Mr. Herriot was a charming, unassuming fellow. Later we visited his veterinary clinic and farm where he practiced before his retirement. My group visited the Royal Veterinary College and the American embassy and had an elegant reception at the Beecham Laboratories Research Center. In my free time I toured palaces, cathedrals, and historic places.

My home is eighty-four years old, ten years my senior. In winter, when the snow is deep and the ploughs are slow, I walk the half mile to work and can see the Verrazano Bridge connecting Staten Island to Brooklyn. I don't know how long I can keep going, but I'd rather not retire. When my friends retire, they seem to age rapidly.

My friend Irene Kraft, who built her own small-animal hospital in White Plains, New York, was a wonderful veterinarian, and we went to all the American Animal Hospital Association meetings together. A while back she had a stroke while spaying a cat and died.

I've made many wonderful friends through veterinary medicine, and my clients keep me aware of what's happening on Staten Island. I'm the island's oldest practicing veterinarian. Still, I can't think of anything in the world I like to do better. My sentimental investment is so profound. ∎

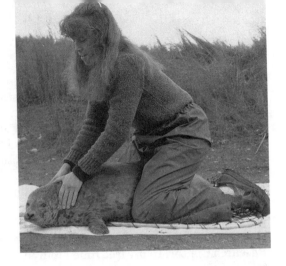

Jessica Porter

THE SUN is bright and warm as the ferry from the mainland cruises steadily through the crystal-blue waters of Puget Sound toward the landing at Friday Harbor, Washington, a small town located on the east side of San Juan Island. The ferry docks, and a young coast guard employee and his wife, carrying an ice chest between them, cross over the ramp. A small gray head with large luminous dark eyes peeks cautiously out of the open chest at the bystanders staring back at it.

Jessica Porter and her husband, George, stride through the crowd, greet the couple, and quickly survey the steel-colored harbor seal pup, an orphan found on a Washington beach. The rescuers carrying him seem both relieved and reluctant to turn over their charge, which they have named Andy.

"He's a good-sized fellow," Porter tells them. "He'll probably be all right. Why don't you come back with us? I'll show you where he'll be staying."

George leaves for his office, a couple of blocks away. The others pile into the Porters' old station wagon and set out for a metal building a few miles away, hidden from the road by dense forest. The building houses the hospital and

living quarters of Wolf Hollow Wildlife Rehabilitation Centre, which Jessica Porter and Judy Carter, her veterinary assistant, founded in 1982. The rescuers carry Andy into the building in his make-shift carrier. Porter, a slight red-haired woman dressed in tank top, jeans, and Reeboks, extracts the slippery baby from his plastic cocoon and places him in the pan of a white metal baby scale.

"Twenty-three pounds," she says with a smile. "That's not too bad. By the time we get these little fellows, they're often so dehydrated that they're down to fourteen pounds. Normally they weigh about twenty-five pounds at birth and can gain up to seventy-five pounds by the time they are three weeks old."

She is working while she talks, and every movement is like choreographed dance—place baby on stainless steel table, attach red rubber stomach tube to sixty-milliliter syringe, fill tube and syringe with formula, pass tube into baby's mouth and over the tongue until he swallows, push syringe plunger with chin and thumb, reload syringe, and repeat the process of propelling life-giving fluids into the orphan.

"We can't simulate a formula to match a seal mother's milk," Porter says.

"Seal milk is about eighty percent fat. We can't even get that much fat in emulsion, so I try to hydrate them with fluids and electrolytes and a suspension of ground fish."

What Porter is really doing is caring for and saving at least a small part of our living planet. Her mission seems almost spiritual but certainly not conventionally religious. In fact, knocking convention seems to be what Jessica Porter is all about.

Porter attended Colorado State University in the 1970s, when agriculture was in its heyday. She explains, "In preveterinary classes, I stood out because I was a liberal hippie when most everyone else seemed to be a conservative cowboy. I enrolled in elective psychology and anthropology courses when most of my classmates opted for 'Feeds and Feeding' and 'Horse Production.' I wanted to doctor reticulated pythons and wolves when others wanted to learn how to get rich in a poodle practice or an equine breeding farm."

With a salary of one hundred dollars a month, Porter is not the richest veterinarian in the world, but she has obviously found her niche in wildlife rehabilitation. Surrounded by eagles, hawks, nesting birds, raccoons, brown-and-white-spotted fawns, harbor seal pups, and various other creatures, Porter expresses her feeling of innate kinship by healing these animals and then setting them free.

■

I think I was born to be a veterinarian, and when I was three years old, I realized on an unconscious level that I owed a debt to animals. It was then that I contracted polio and nearly died.

Although I stayed in the hospital for many long months, I gradually recovered enough to be released for home care. I was an only child, and I think my parents were unable to cope with such a seriously ill baby. While I was hospitalized, they started to distance themselves from me and the situation.

When I came home, I was very lonely, as well as handicapped. I turned to the family dog, which was a Great Dane. Dragging heavy leg braces with me, I pulled myself erect and literally climbed up that dog, and she would patiently stand there and let me crawl all over her. The two of us—human and animal—made a connection, and that trust and unconditional love helped me to survive.

In certain ways you might say I had a privileged upbringing. I was born in Cleveland and grew up in New York City, where my father was an executive in a large brewery. When I was eight years old, I was sent to a boarding school in Surrey, England. I graduated from that school ten years later.

There was no agony over what to do with my life after high school graduation, because I had decided to become a zoo veterinarian. I made that decision in the third grade after I read a book titled *Circus Doctor*, which sort of pulled all of my interests together.

The hard part in the late sixties was finding a veterinary school that offered any kind of a program in zoo-animal medicine. I finally decided to go to Colorado State University at Fort Collins, Colorado, because it was one of two veterinary schools in the world to offer a preceptorship at a zoo.

It was total culture shock when I moved to Colorado. I had come from a cosmopolitan background, and at that time, Fort Collins was very rural. The veterinary school placed heavy emphasis on large-animal medicine, and the campus as a whole catered to students majoring in animal science and the other agricultural disciplines.

The cowboys ran roughshod over parts of the campus and town and often harassed hippies who ventured onto what the cowboys considered their turf. I majored in preveterinary medicine, which was part of that territory, and I stood out like chalk on a blackboard. I didn't wear cowboy boots, I spoke with an English accent, and I looked like a hippie. If I had majored in anthropology or sociology instead of preveterinary medicine, I probably wouldn't have been noticed.

I met my future husband, George, a native of Colorado, at CSU, and we lived together while I completed my preprofessional courses. When I realized that my chances of being accepted by the veterinary school would be better as a Colorado resident, we decided to get married. In those days, a female could assume her husband's residency.

However, when I applied to veterinary school, I faced additional discrimination—because I was female and because I was married. I was supposed to feel responsible for taking the place of a man, especially when my husband might move and insist that I follow him.

I was turned down by the veterinary school two years in a row. In the meantime, I obtained a B.S. degree in microbiology and took the first two years of the veterinary curriculum for noncredit. I audited the veterinary school classes and asked the teachers to hold my grades. I proved that I could do the work by making an A or a B in each class, and I was finally legitimately admitted into the College of Veterinary Medicine after completing the first two years. I was the first married woman accepted by the veterinary school. I differed from my classmates because my main interest was wildlife medicine. I did two preceptorships back-to-back at the Denver zoo because nobody else was interested in going there. Today there is a waiting list for this kind of training. But in those days, zoo medicine was strange enough, and an interest in wildlife was considered off-the-wall. Many considered me strange anyway, so my interest in wild animals seemed to confirm their suspicions.

My veterinary school professors knew little and seemed to care even less about exotic species. Today the College of Veterinary Medicine at CSU has a raptor center, and the emphasis on zoo and wildlife medicine has greatly increased. But back then, I was the wildlife and zoo program. If a snake or lion came in, I dealt with it. I was allowed to use the neurology ward for my patients, and I often upset the neurology professor because I tended to take over his ward.

I remember when a fellow student who now owns a lucrative small-animal practice in Hawaii told me that I could never make a living working with wild animals. I told him that I didn't care, and he responded that I had to care because I had to eat. We were good friends but had totally opposite goals.

After graduation from veterinary school, I worked for a short time at the Denver zoo and the North American Wildlife Center near Golden, Colorado.

While at the wildlife center, I set up a refuge for wolves. For the most part, we took pet wolves and retrained them to be wild. We kept a core pack of wolves just to train the others how to behave like their species. It was common for people to buy the cute little furry fellows when they were pups and then give them up when they grew into large unruly adolescents. We had cases of three- and four-year-old wolves that had been kept in a three-by-five-foot cage for their entire lives. When they were put into a larger enclosure, they still paced three-by-five. We had about a 50 percent success rate, meaning we released half to the wild and had to destroy the other half because they couldn't learn to be wolves.

The last year George and I lived in Colorado, I taught a course in human physiology and sexuality at CSU, along with my work at the zoo and wildlife center. During this time, George completed a master's degree in computer engineering.

George and I have been divorced twice and married three

times. We've always kept our marriage as a renewable contract. During the long period that we've known each other, I've changed and had different goals, and he has changed and had different goals. We stay together when we're happy doing that, and we part when we're not. We've lived that way for a long time and have always come back together.

One of my goals in veterinary school was to pursue a residency at a large zoo following graduation. The opportunity came to become a resident at the London Zoo, and I left Colorado and went back to what I consider home, England. It was one of those things that I thought I wanted—to be a staff veterinarian at a large zoological park.

There were some good times—short trips to participate in wildlife research in Venezuela and Africa—but for the most part, I became disenchanted with becoming a permanent member of a zoo staff. All I really wanted to do was work with animals; yet it seemed that all I was doing was paper shuffling and administrative work. At age thirty-one, I had a mid-life crisis. Life became very difficult, and everything I tried to do took monumental effort. I'd wake up in the mornings depressed, thinking that I was wasting my life. I wasn't really doing anything to help animals.

I finally realized that I had to relax, open my mind and spirit to the higher powers, and allow things to happen when the time was right. Two or three weeks later, I went to a meeting in Seattle about orcas [killer whales] presented by the Whale Museum in Friday Harbor, Washington. A week after that, I was offered a full-time job as educational coordinator at the museum.

Whale and seal research piqued my interest, so I accepted the job and moved to Friday Harbor, a small island town. I have lived in Friday Harbor ever since, and I love it here. The island where I live is less than fifty-six square miles, and some folks find that living in such a confined space is claustrophobic. These same people get upset if the ferries are backed up and they can't get to the mainland or from the mainland home, and they usually move away from here. But for me, the island is perfect. The mainland has too much stimulation: noise, lights, traffic, and people. The only way people can live with all that distraction is to block most of it out. Once you dampen your senses, you also kill part of your spirit. It is important for me to use all of my senses without feeling constantly bombarded.

After a while, the residents of the island got to know me and encouraged me to set up a veterinary practice. I had never practiced, so I thought that I ought to consider it. However, I didn't have a Washington license and the thought of taking the state board really made me hesitant about making definite plans. I had been out of school several years by this time and didn't know how much I remembered about domestic animals. I knew I would do great if the test emphasized killer whales, wolves, and golden eagles, but frankly, veterinary boards do not place an emphasis on exotic animals. I took the board, forgot about it, and went to Alaska for several weeks.

This is obviously a small town, because the townspeople knew before I did that I had passed the board. The first I knew of it was through a newspaper clipping from the local newspaper that a friend sent to me in Alaska. The article said something like "Dr. Jessica Porter recently received her license to practice veterinary medicine in the state of Washington and will be opening a veterinary practice in Friday Harbor in the near future."

I came back home and rented a small house on the main street and set up a mixed practice. I always said that if I ever owned anything, I'd name it after my very best friends. The hospital was called Wolf Hollow Veterinary Clinic.

Wolf Hollow was a 1930s-style practice because most people around here couldn't afford high-tech services. And the surprising thing is that it's possible to keep animals alive without a CAT scan. It's even possible to keep some animals alive without blood tests when the owners won't consent to them. My practice was about 50 percent large and 50 percent small animals. I saw everything, including dogs, cats, rabbits, birds, goats, sheep, pigs, horses, cattle, and llamas.

In addition, I took in injured wildlife. Wolf Hollow Veterinary Clinic and Wolf Hollow Wildlife Rehabilitation Centre more or less existed jointly. At one time, I had four seal pups, six fawns, several eagles, lots of raccoons, and the private practice, all on an eighth of an acre in the middle of town. It was insane, and I finally became aware that I couldn't handle it all. It wasn't fair to clients or to the wildlife. By this time, I had all the federal and state licenses that I needed to do wildlife rehabilitation, and I thought that donations would help support the work. After six years in practice, I sold it for the huge sum of eight hundred dollars to devote full time to my wild animals.

Finding a place to do my work was my first priority, so I put a simple ad in the local newspaper that read, "Wolf Hollow Wildlife Rehabilitation Centre needs property." I received a call from someone who had forty acres that were secluded but close to town. They offered to lease the land to me for one dollar a year. Thus, Wolf Hollow moved to its current location. I have found that when what we are doing is right, the universe opens up and supplies what we need.

Wolf Hollow has come a long way in two years. The building, which now houses George's and my living quarters and the hospital, was once a metal shell with a dirt floor. When we moved here, we had no heat, no electricity, and no running water. We moved a trailer next to the building and went to work. First we poured a concrete floor and added electrical wiring. Then we renovated the building to accommodate a kitchen and a treatment room downstairs, and a bedroom, a bath, and a nursery upstairs. When we have intensive-care babies, I roll out of bed every two hours to feed them; it helps to have the nursery close by.

People seemed to come from everywhere to help. Glenn Thielberg, an Air Force retiree and former veterinary client, came to Wolf Hollow to bury his old dog Kip on the property and has been living here and helping out ever since. Local residents, usually four or five at a time, volunteer services, and we now have college students—wildlife interns—who come and stay up to two months with us. We furnish these young people with a place to stay while they do a wildlife project for which they receive credit through their local universities. We also offer a wildlife preceptorship for veterinary students from Washington State University and Colorado State University. People see what I do here, and they want to be a part of it.

Judy Carter, who worked for me when I owned the veterinary practice, George, and I are considered staff at Wolf Hollow. We are each paid a salary of one hundred dollars per month. There is no money in wildlife rehabilitation, and most veterinarians who do it must have a secondary source of income. However, I have no needs that are not being met. I pay no rent. I buy all of my clothes except my running shoes at garage sales. Some of the things that society places such value on—new cars, movies, and going out to dinner—aren't necessary for me.

But we do need things for the animals. Until 1987, Wolf Hollow, which is a tax-exempt nonprofit enterprise, depended solely on unsolicited donations. We wanted a better way of getting the word out about our work and needs, so last year my husband quit his job as a computer engineer to become a full-time fund-raiser for the center.

George has begun a campaign to raise four hundred thousand dollars. We recently bought the property and want to build a new hospital, a 108-by-40-foot flight cage for the eagles and hawks, a concrete pool for the seals, and a walk-in freezer to store bulk food. Just feeding the animals can be a monumental task. Each year we feed thousands of pounds of fish to the baby seals, otters, seabirds, and other animals. We have three donated freezers, and we can often buy fish cheaper in season and save it for later. I've also learned to scrounge. I pick up perfectly good produce that the grocery stores in town normally throw out, and I feed it to the animals.

George's work is definitely paying off. One of his efforts is a newsletter titled *Wild Times,* which is mailed to nearly two thousand interested people and organizations. As more people hear about us, they send in injured wildlife or make donations of time, supplies, or money. Our rescue calls have increased from approximately 10 in 1982 to more than 250 in 1988. And these numbers don't reflect the cases that can be resolved without bringing in an animal. For example, a person calls after picking up a fawn that the mother doe carefully left hidden while she went to graze. That person would be told to take the fawn back to the same spot, leave it, and check on it after twilight. Ninety percent of the time, Mom comes back to retrieve her offspring. And if she doesn't, we do.

We've received great publicity from television programs about the center that have been aired on all the major stations in Portland and Seattle. We even appeared in a television program titled "Love around the World," which aired in Tokyo. The Japanese producers found us through a magazine article about Wolf Hollow, and that's how it goes—someone reads about or sees us, and that leads to the next article or program.

Wolf Hollow's mission is threefold: rehabilitate wildlife, provide education about wildlife, and research the habitat, needs, and ways of wild animals. Our rehabilitative goals include responding to calls about injured or orphaned wildlife, providing animals with shelter and medical treatment, and returning animals that have recuperated to the wild. We receive calls about animals that need help from state and federal wildlife officials, police personnel, port managers, other rehabilitators, and private citizens. Animals we see routinely include raccoons, fox, otters, deer, elephant seals, harbor seals, and all kinds of birds, including eagles, hawks, owls, migratory birds, and songbirds.

Sometimes things seem to work simply and smoothly. I recently received a call about a young elephant seal that had beached herself. A couple of assistants held her down while I removed a shaft that was protruding through her lip. She seemed all right otherwise, and we were able to release her into the water. Other times, nothing seems to work. Little harbor seals often come in so dehydrated that it is impossible to save them, or we lose the baby raccoons to parvovirus or starvation.

My veterinary medical background is essential for what I do, but I am trying now to be more of a rehabilitator and less of a veterinarian. Too much medicine adds stress to these animals, just at a time when they don't need it. I never use antibiotics unless it is absolutely necessary. I have seen so many fawns suffering from bloat and other abnormalities of the rumen [a stomach compartment], which were treated with antibiotics by well-meaning but unknowing veterinarians.

Other caring people may try to raise an orphan wild animal but, in the process, ruin the animal for leading the life nature intended. They are not doing an animal a favor by humanizing it. At about two weeks of age, birds of prey will imprint on whoever is feeding it, and if the baby bird imprints on a species different from its own, it will not breed or know what it's supposed to be. We use an eagle puppet when we feed young bald eagles. The puppets are not fancy, just something that looks like an eagle with a black body, white head, and yellow beak. With mammals, it's not so much that they fix on humans but that they don't have one of their own species to identify with. If you raise two raccoons together, they will know they are raccoons.

Once our wild babies are weaned, we use aversion therapy to teach them to fear humans. We make loud noises with a dishpan and a spoon. I may take my two dogs, Aero and Hector, with me around the fawns, so they will associate humans with the obnoxious barking of dangerous animals. I also teach trap aversion. I don't want one of my animals to be caught in a leg-hold trap.

I keep some animals that are humanized, for teaching purposes. I have had Arthur, a boa constrictor, for seventeen years. He's twenty-one now and will probably outlive me. I adopted Arthur when he had reconstructive surgery on his nose after being attacked by a rat. Then he developed mouthrot, and I used to carry him around with me in a pouch, so I could medicate him every few hours. Arthur is a real gentleman, and I take him to schools to teach children that reptiles are not scary creatures.

Harold is a blind long-eared owl that was found here on the island. Long-eared owls aren't supposed to live here, but a local nesting pair must have produced Harold. Harold loves the attention he receives in the classroom and is a very good teacher. Angus the raccoon and Pogo the otter are also great classroom performers. Regardless of how friendly and cute these animals are, they should never be kept as pets. This is something I emphasize to audiences. Angus and Pogo belong in the wild with others of their species, and Pogo was recently set free.

Teaching is one of the priorities at Wolf Hollow, and we enjoy working with young people because they hear you with such open minds. I edited a children's book for the Whale Museum titled *Gentle Giants of the Sea.*

One of our goals in working with adults is to present alternative ways of thinking. In an effort to reach out to adult audiences and educate them about environmental issues, I teach a class called "Environmental and Wildlife Awareness" at the local branch of the community college.

You can accomplish quite a lot and have an impact on lives in a small community. I was one of three people instrumental in starting the Islands Oil Spill Organization to protect our local islands against oil spills. The thrust of the organization is oil containment and bird rescue. Our organization became the prototype for many island communities within the state of Washington.

I have maintained my affiliation with the Whale Museum by serving as its staff veterinarian. If a marine mammal dies and washes up on shore, I work with the museum's scientists to try to determine why the animal was stranded and why it died. I will perform a necropsy on dead animals and consult about treatment for sick animals. This type of collaboration helps both Wolf Hollow and the Whale Museum. Plus, we share a permit from the National Marine Fisheries Service that allows us to do rehabilitative work for marine mammals.

Wolf Hollow's research goals are as follows: to learn more about the habitat as it exists now for each species in our area, to discover threats to animals and to the habitat, to invent the best medical treatment and rehabilitation facilities, and to learn from individual animals. We never perform any experiment that might be considered intrusive or harmful to individual animals.

We have so much to learn from animals. Every pet I had when I was growing up taught me to love unconditionally and to care. The little acts of altruism between wild animals are so pure.

These creatures have no ulterior motives, and that's why they are so good for children and older people. I've taken animals into nursing homes, and the place totally changes. There is such pure communication between animals and people.

I didn't see this basic connection as much in a traditional dog-and-cat practice because animals often take on the psychopathology of their owners. Essentially, they aren't animals anymore. However, every once in a while, you run into an animal that really looks at you and makes contact. You know that you've made a connection with a part of the earth, and that's a liberating and peaceful feeling.

It is hard to let the animals that come into our lives go sometimes. I've had to deal with the loss and frustration of watching animals I've worked with die. I used to think that I was going to save all of them. That was part of what we were taught in veterinary school. Our function was to save lives, and when we couldn't, we had failed somehow.

As part of my evolution, I took courses on the topic of death and dying. In dealing with the death of an animal, you go through the same stages of grief—denial, anger, guilt, depression, and finally acceptance—that Dr. Elisabeth Kubler-Ross outlined for people. I have felt all of these emotions. Why did that seal pup come in just to die five minutes later and subject me to the pain of its death? It could have died in the wild, and I wouldn't have felt the loss.

A friend of mine helped me accept that certain animals are here for only a short period of time; regardless of the length of time, each animal teaches me something. The lesson may be scientific or medical—I learn a new procedure or treatment—or it may be spiritual. Sometimes it seems that the animal came into my life simply to say thank you and leave. I've learned to let go. It's not our place to grab hold when it's time for an animal to go to the next dimension, whatever we as individuals believe that next dimension to be.

Emotions such as anger and depression, which are part of the grieving process, are also evident when individuals or whole communities feel powerless. That seems to be the situation at most oil spills because the affected community feels victimized by the disaster.

I have been a contract veterinarian for the International Bird Rescue Research Center in Berkeley, California. This organization works with oil companies to provide help for animals affected by oil spills. I spent nine weeks during the spring of 1989 at the Exxon spill in Valdez, Alaska.

The situation at Valdez has taught us how fragile a pristine environment really is. The authorities thought the oil pipeline was safe, but the pipeline had a history of only ten years, which really isn't all that long. After the spill, the local residents felt raped. They also felt invaded by the people from Exxon, the press, and the people who came to clean up. They needed to heal, and they needed to take part in cleaning their own environment in order to heal.

The economic aspects at Valdez were obvious. Most of the locals, the Indians and fishers, had lost their incomes for the year or years. However, the social implications were less obvious. There was an increase in wife beating, child abuse, and alcoholism. People who feel victimized and helpless strike out. They have to find something or someone they can have power over.

I don't think that the Prince William sound is permanently destroyed, but it is compromised and will be for a good decade. If a corporation is big enough, it's very difficult to make it assume anything but financial responsibility. Exxon didn't lose money on the spill; it just raised oil prices. Every person who buys a tank of gas is paying for it.

We have got to educate people to take one less trip into town or to walk instead of drive. We cannot continue to depend upon fossil fuels for energy. We cannot afford a disposable society.

Each individual in this country has a lot of power, and we can use that power to save our environment. We can go to the town council meeting and write to legislators and mobilize our neighbors to do so, too. We can say that we care about the environment and about our endangered species, like the bald eagle, and we can vote for politicians who are ecologically aware. The squeaky wheel gets attention, and it doesn't matter if a person lives in New York City or San Juan Island.

It's a question of whether we succumb to greed or evolve past greed for the good of the planet. If we can't save the wildlife, we can't save ourselves. Living creatures all have the same requirements for life—clean air, clean water, clean food, and space in which to live. If I can educate one or two people a day or week to care for the animals and to care for the earth, it spreads by the ripple effect.

But I don't know if we can change fast enough. We are continuing to pollute the environment. The hole in the ozone layer in our atmosphere appears to be growing. Acid rain is ruining many watersheds on the East Coast, and we are destroying rain forests all over the world.

We are accepting pollution without a fight. The soil in many areas of Colorado and other western states is contaminated with radioactive waste. People are buying food poisoned by toxins and feeding it to their families. The cancer rate in children has tripled in the last thirty years, and there's got to be a reason for that.

People adapt and put up with these things. We may be adapting too easily and giving up on some of these important issues. We can demand clean air, clean water, and clean food.

I decided early on to live my life according to my convictions. I am a vegetarian because I believe it is morally wrong to eat animals. We can get all of the protein that we need without killing an animal to do it, and we would be healthier in the long run.

I wouldn't do anything to an animal that I wouldn't do to myself, and I certainly wouldn't do what is done to cattle in a slaughterhouse. A reverence for life starts at a very basic level. If you can shoot a bird for the sport of it, you might be able to shoot a person of another color, religion, or belief for the sport of it. More people are saying on a grass-roots level that whaling is wrong, that fur coats are wrong, and that eating meat is wrong.

George and I have elected to remain childless. Not having children is another way to save the earth. If every couple would have only one child, we could halve our overpopulation problem in one generation. Overpopulation, which equates to lack of food and lack of space, is the greatest problem facing the world today.

I went to India in the early sixties. I saw a man, his pregnant wife, and six children on the side of the road. They had one piece of bread among them and were obviously starving. It doesn't take a lot of education to know that the more children you have, the smaller the piece of bread becomes.

If you put too many rats in a cage, they become stressed and start eating their babies. Child abuse has risen to astronomical highs. That's what we are doing in a sense—"eating our babies."

I have had to learn to deal with stress in my own life. I go from 7 A.M. until 11 P.M. seven days a week until the wild babies are gone in November. This schedule is teaching me to deal with stress on a day-to-day basis. I relieve stress by meditating and running.

The running has become a rebirthing process for me. After I had polio, I was told that I would never be able to run. I believed that for thirty-five years. Then George encouraged me to start running. I told him that I couldn't do it because I had lost my proprioceptive senses. However, I started and found that I'm good at it. George is my coach, and we run together. I run 5 miles every day and 10 miles on weekends. Next year, I plan to run in a 146-mile ultramarathon. The Badwater Run from Death Valley to Mount Whitney in California is a goal I've set for myself.

Someday I hope to have another chief wildlife rehabilitator on the Wolf Hollow staff. I would then have more time to pursue my other goals, such as competitive running, oil-spill rescue, and research. I am a person who needs goals to center my focus on. Because my goal to become a veterinarian was well defined, the barriers I experienced getting into veterinary school only increased my convictions.

Although women of my era were discouraged from pursuing veterinary medicine as a career, I think my gender has been a professional asset. For example, I have received a lot of publicity because I am small, female, and, until recently, young. People enjoy watching a very small person working with a large animal. Visitors loved it when I wrestled an alligator at the zoo. If I had been a six-foot-tall man, they probably wouldn't have noticed.

Women have a responsibility to their gender just like all minorities have a responsibility to their group. When you are breaking ground, you are more heavily scrutinized and open to criticism, and it doesn't matter if you are African-American or Hispanic or female. Women have a tremendous amount of power—mental power, intuitive power, and spiritual power—if they only know how to use it. My power comes from being a woman, from the animals, from being grounded in the earth, and from being open to the universe.

My ultimate goals have always been those projects the universe hands over to me to deal with, so I don't know what my future direction will be or what the universe has in store for me. ■

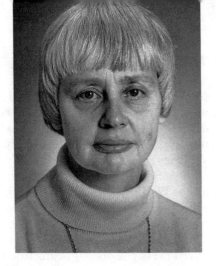

Sandra Siwe

ON the Serengeti, where the average tourist is clothed in abrasion-resistant khaki that blends with land and bush, the chief warden easily picks out the vibrant orange of an Illini T-shirt and is quietly amused and relieved that Sandra Siwe is, for the moment, safe. Even in uncivilized Africa, where humans are intruders, Siwe is a nonconformist.

Siwe graduated from the University of Illinois in 1963, when there were only two small-animal hospitals in Champaign-Urbana. Today there are eleven small-animal hospitals, and Siwe is a co-owner of two of them and of one satellite clinic. She has practiced small-animal medicine since graduation, except for three years as a resident student and teacher in anesthesiology at the University of Illinois. Those three years convinced Siwe that her real love was practice.

Siwe keeps her enthusiasm alive by scheduling sufficient time away from work. Touring with small groups of serious naturalists, she studies wildlife in remote areas of Africa, South America, Australia, New Zealand, and the Antarctic. In this off time, hardly spent relaxing, she becomes an explorer and a risk taker.

■

If I could live without the financial support of my animal hospitals, I would flee to Africa and settle in Botswana, where the land is 80 to 90 percent desert—the Kalahari—and, during the rainy season, swamp. There's no irrigation, no paved roads, as of six years ago, and only subsistence farming. With very little human encroachment, animal life abounds. Places unseen by humans may still exist.

As things are, I pay incredible sums of money to live three weeks in Botswana in a remote tent camp. There supplies are flown in one year ahead, dinner plates are hot off the coals, and scorpions play on the tablecloth.

I don't need civilization. Life here in my house in Champaign, Illinois, is so artificial. I can live without a microwave and other gadgets that plug in and a telephone. I, who am a slave to the phone in my job, find Botswana a wonderful place with no phones.

Since 1977 I have been to Africa five times. I've toured game reserves in Kenya, the Serengeti, Tanzania, South Africa, and Botswana, and I've looked at the relics and geology of Egypt. In Africa I want to get as close to the animals and the land as possible. I want to feel the heat, the dust, the insects. I want to have the same intimate contact with the environment that the animals have. The number of animals is always declining. A rhinoceros is so rare that if a tour guide spots one, he or she radios its location to all the other guides in the area. In no time, Land-Rovers full of tourists converge on the poor beast. Poachers kill rhinos for their horns and elephants for ivory. You can't blame the natives. They are so poor, and animal parts and pelts have big price tags. Of course, there are laws against poaching, but it's not possible to police such large land areas.

If the last elephant died tomorrow, not many people would be affected. But the chance to experience an elephant would be gone. If you've never experienced their intelligence or watched elephants in a herd care for each other and their young, you cannot perceive the tragedy of this loss. This is why I feel an incredible urgency to return to Africa and experience the animals before they vanish.

There is nothing like encountering an elephant for the first time, while sleeping in a dark tent. Because I was the only woman in the tent camp, the guides insured my privacy by giving me a tent in an isolated corner. At bedtime, I was handed a chamber pot and told to stay in my tent to avoid wild animals that wandered through camp at night. Jolted awake by loud stamping, ripping, and crunching, I heard the rumbling of an enormous ruminant stomach and realized an elephant was uprooting the succulent ornamental plants outside my tent. Distracted by hunger, he crashed into my tent, then panicked and stampeded into the darkness. In the morning I found a jovial group of native guides gathered outside, studying the prints.

"Did you have a little trouble last night?" they asked.

"Yes," I told them, "but I stayed in the tent!"

I've watched a herd of elephants approach a water hole at dusk while the lead cow, as appointed guardian, circled nervously. In a small dugout canoe, I've drifted among oversize hippos soaking in a muddy, dung-filled river and watched, amazed, when my guide quenched his thirst with a handful of river water. I could never go to these places unharmed without my native guide. These native Africans are remarkable people. Self-educated, they can identify a large number of bird and animal species and often speak several foreign languages. They aren't allowed to carry guns, so they must know the habits of the wild animals intimately and be able to sense danger.

My wilderness adventures are absolutely essential to my enjoyment of life. I like practice, but the day-to-day humdrum routine eventually dulls my mind. I become stale and lose interest in learning new things. I return from these trips energized. Practice is fun again. Not everyone is like this. My clinic partner, John Lykins, comes back from a luxury cruise exhausted. "God, I hated it," he says. He gets his high in a different way.

At home, in my university city, my life needs routine. I am typically up at 6 A.M. I skip breakfast, except for coffee, but the boys—my bloodhound and springer spaniel—insist on theirs. I am a slave to my dogs and look after their every need. Before I leave for work, there is usually an undisturbed hour to catch up on bills or chores or professional reading or to browse through *Smithsonian* or *Natural History* magazine, where I get many of my travel ideas. The dogs go to the animal hospital with me and rest in cages until lunch.

My partner and I start work at about eight. I met John when we both worked for the University of Illinois, and we decided to build the hospital together. I do surgery all morning while John sees clients. I like surgery and encourage referrals from neighboring veterinarians. They know I taught anesthesiology at the veterinary college, so they give me their overweight, weak-heart, poor-risk patients.

At noon I feed and exercise my dogs, then drive to the local YMCA for a twenty-minute swim. This is necessary therapy for my left shoulder joint. In 1985 an inflammation from some unknown cause froze my left shoulder joint and made that arm essentially useless. I interrogated four doctors before I found a man who believed my arm could regain normal function. It took a year of pills and exercise, but now I have greater range of motion in my left arm than my right. Still, I must exercise constantly. I'm in a group of YMCA regulars who show up on schedule year after year. If I miss a day, everyone asks where I've been.

I'm back at the animal hospital by three and see clients until six. My friends know they can find me at home in the evenings. My social life is pretty low-key, an occasional dinner or play at the university.

Neither John nor I take after-hours emergency calls. I hire veterinary students from the university to screen our calls, and if an animal needs immediate attention, they call one of our part-time professional staff members. We have no trouble hiring graduate students. Recently we had one student working on a master's degree in parasitology and one on a Ph.D. in physiology. They are eager for the money and the clinic experience. Presently I work a four-and-one-half-day week, taking Wednesday off and working Saturday morning.

John and I emphasize personal service and tend to build close working friendships with our clients. As the area grows, we grow. The population of Champaign-Urbana is up to one hundred thousand, and six new veterinary hospitals have opened since I graduated in 1963. In 1984 we opened a one-person outpatient clinic just six miles away. In 1989, construction of our new full-service hospital in Urbana was finished. John and I will stay at our original hospital in the cornfields of Champaign.

I have the only hospital in the area that does not schedule appointments except for surgery or radiographs. When I graduated, most animal hospitals didn't make appointments, and my clients like the old way best. My clients are well informed on the advances in veterinary medicine, and most are willing to pay for good service, so we accommodate them. Not only do we send critical cases to the university for state-of-the-art tests and monitoring, but we've also designed a preventive-care program that our clients follow enthusiastically. This includes vaccinations, stool checks, heartworm tests, dentistry, geriatric profiles, and nutrition and behavioral counseling. We look for problems before they get out of hand.

It seems that I see more long-term, incurable conditions than I used to, like diabetes mellitus, low thyroid or high thyroid, and skin allergies. In the sixties if a veterinarian told clients that their dog had an allergy, he or she would have been called a quack. Now allergies are common. I never hesitate to tell people they are dealing with a persistent problem that has no cure. Once they understand this, they stop spending money on new opinions, and we work together to keep their dog as close to normal as possible.

Of course, being neighbors with the veterinary college is a big advantage. The college has the equipment and workforce to provide care that no small-animal hospital can offer. For example, I had a nine-year-old diabetic Saint Bernard collapse three hours after I did surgery to remove her infected uterus. The owners rushed her to the university clinics, where the staff monitored her blood sugar values and injected insulin around the clock for three days.

Another case was a twelve-year-old Siberian husky hit by a snowplow, with compound fractures of both front legs. The students and professors put her legs together with bone plates and wires and monitored her until she decided to live. By fourteen years of age this husky had survived two more university surgeries, both to remove a persistent tumor from her nasal sinus. A husky's average life span is twelve years, but the owners of this dog willingly spent more than five thousand dollars to keep her alive. This tells me that pets today are as important as ever, and people will pay for good health care.

I also see an increase in behavior problems among pet dogs and cats. The average dog owner is looking for a pleasant companion and really has no desire to dominate and direct the dog's life. This lack of direction and discipline unnerves many dogs, especially the large breeds. They display all sorts of aberrant behavior, from destruction to aggression. I believe women veterinarians often identify these problems before male veterinarians. It is more in the woman's nature to empathize with the pet owner. Men know that pets are thought of as family members, but they feel less comfortable than the women in these emotional situations.

I have two dogs of my own that I treat like family. Love me, love my dogs. Ask my friends. My new Caravan already smells like a dog, with nose marks on the windows and the cargo area full of dog crates, chew bones, and leashes. Even my house is dog-proof, with sheets over the furniture. I collect antique Russian and Turkish samovars, the only indestructible object I can place on a low table. There's no way a wagging tail can destroy these heavy bronze tea servers.

Rameses is my sixth bloodhound. Stomach bloat is common in this breed and can kill the dogs at an early age. When Rameses was young, I taught him how to track. This is a wonderful sport for both of us. The dog must follow a particular human scent on a mile course that twists through briars, woods, ravines, sand, and swamp. Cross scents are laid to confuse the dog. At trail's end, the dog's only reward is a glove belonging to the person who laid the trail.

In my opinion, bloodhounds have a one-neuron brain that is easily overloaded. Even with their superior nose, hours of repetition and reinforcement are necessary to train them, but once they catch on, they never forget. When Rameses learned to track, he hit all trails at top speed. In competition a dog is introduced to the scent between two metal flagpoles fifteen yards apart. Most dogs lie down and sniff the grass until the scent is clear in their head. Not Rameses! As soon as he saw the flags, he started howling and zoomed through the start head high, nose full of scent. Hanging on to a forty-foot leash, I had to follow. If I dropped the leash, we were disqualified. Rameses has won all the top awards. I have the scars to prove it.

Now I'm teaching Sage, my two-year-old springer to track. He catches on much more quickly than Rameses, but he's such a show-off. During competition we're followed by judges and a small gallery of spectators. Sage likes to leap into the air unexpectedly to view his audience. I train year-round in all weather, except hot summer.

I'm an animal maniac. Before I even knew what veterinary medicine was, I wanted to take care of sick animals. I kept every kind of pet that would fit in our house and yard in the Milwaukee suburbs. I must have been a tomboy. I played outdoors all day, fishing and climbing trees. I'd round up friends, and we'd ride our bikes to the edge of town, which was much closer in those days. We'd catch horses grazing in a pasture and scramble onto their bare backs.

My parents were very forward-thinking for the 1940s and 1950s and encouraged my free spirit. My father was a big-city stockbroker, a high-pressure job. My mother never went to college but managed our family as well as any corporate president. Dad gave her his paycheck, and she paid the bills. In the evening, Dad stayed with my brother and me while Mom worked part-time. My brother was seven years younger than me.

On career day at high school, no veterinarian showed up, so I tagged along with classmates who wanted to be medical doctors. We were taken to the local hospital and allowed to watch an autopsy. I'll never forget the corpse—a 250-pound woman who had died from a gallstone. The pathologist sawed through her ribs and skull and showed us every organ in her body.

That night at dinner, I shared my excitement with my family, regaling them with gory details while stuffing my mouth with food. Nobody else ate. But my parents never interrupted or stifled my enthusiasm.

After high school, I attended the University of Wisconsin at Milwaukee for three years. I needed only two years of preveterinary credits, but there were so many tantalizing courses that I stayed an extra year.

Wisconsin did not have a veterinary college, so I applied to more than a dozen out-of-state universities. My counselor kept telling me, "Even with your high grades, no school is going to take you, because you are a woman." Unfortunately, he spoke some truth. Two eastern schools told me to forget it because I was out-of-state and a woman. Michigan wanted one year of practical farm experience, but the University of Illinois sent me an application. I filled it out and was accepted, pending a personal interview.

The morning of my interview, my father announced he was going with me. I couldn't talk him out of this terrible idea. I was twenty-one, and I had to introduce my father to the dean and faculty members on the review committee. Dad let them ask me one question, then he took charge. He wanted to know how they were going to make me happy. After graduation, what sort of salary could they guarantee? He was unremitting as he delved into every aspect of student training and how the instructors would cultivate my abilities. I wanted to put a bag over my head. Finally the dean offered to give us a personal tour of the basic science building and the animal clinics. The large-animal clinic was under construction, but my father wanted to see the locker facilities for women. Satisfied that they would be complete when I arrived, Dad cut the tour short. All the way home in the car, I yelled at my father to make certain he knew he had ruined my life.

The next day a letter of acceptance came. Now, when I think back, I can laugh. After my four years were complete and I, with my parents, passed through the receiving line for veterinary graduates, the dean and professors remembered my dad.

Near the end of my junior year in veterinary college, I married Tom Siwe, a music major, working on his master's degree. All my friends liked Tom. He was quiet and easygoing, a good contrast to my explosive personality.

After graduation, I interviewed with small-animal practitioners in the Chicago area. When men told me I was worth less money, I told them bluntly that I wasn't. In those days I must have seemed very brazen, but that is my natural way. Dr. Harry Cook, a veterinarian in Morton Grove, finally hired me as his first associate. He towered a powerful six feet four and liked to roar harmlessly when things went wrong. I'm sure he chose me for my guts. Included in the deal was a roomy apartment above the animal hospital. Tom stayed in Champaign to finish his master's. I practiced such long hours that there wasn't time to miss him. Still, I was lonely. By the time Tom arrived, he had to share our bedroom with a springer spaniel and a bloodhound puppy.

After six years working with Dr. Cook in Morton Grove, I followed Tom back to the University of Illinois. He had been appointed head of the music department, and I joined a veterinary research group. We studied ways to control blood parasites in livestock. I hated research. All our studies depended on a disembodied tube of blood. There was no animal contact.

After one year studying blood parasites, I accepted a residency at the veterinary college in small-animal anesthesia. I was handling animals again, teaching students, and earning credits toward a master's in anesthesiology. This took place between 1969 and 1973, and I was the only woman on the staff—just me and the secretaries.

After a while I knew enough to teach my colleagues in practice. At seminars I reviewed the two new injectable anesthetics, xylazine and Ketamine. I talked about nonrebreathing systems for animals under fifteen pounds. I demonstrated small induction chambers for cats and rabbits. I stressed warming the animal during surgery and using reliable heart and respiratory monitors. I developed a model crash cart containing all the drugs and equipment immediately needed in cardiac or respiratory arrest.

Talking to seasoned practitioners was a nice boost to my ego, but it couldn't compensate for the ever-tightening university regulations. Against my will, I was slowly being molded. I found John Lykins, a longtime friend, just finishing his Ph.D. in immunology. We decided to escape together by building our own small-animal hospital. The doors opened in 1973, and I was back in practice, never regretting that I left school without completing requirements for a master's degree.

As much as I love practice, I can't let it fill my whole life. There is too much to discover. I take full advantage of a large junior college near the animal hospital to learn how to identify precious gemstones and I study constellations in the sky with teenagers in my astronomy class. I even built a telescope to measure mountains on the moon. Now friends ask me to buy jewels for them when I travel abroad, and I have knowing conversations with diamond experts in South Africa.

In 1979, when I was just past forty years of age, divorced, and living alone with my two dogs, I suddenly understood that life is temporary. This concept began with a common head cold that steadily grew worse. After a week of self-treatment, I consulted the Champaign doctors, who tested all parts of me and pronounced me fit. I grew weaker and burned with a constant 105-degree fever. Finally I stopped work. Convinced I was dying, I called my brother in Milwaukee. He drove through the night to reach me and rushed me to a Milwaukee hospital. I have dreamlike memories of being wheeled down corridors on a gurney. They diagnosed mycoplasma pneumonia, a bacteria that responds almost immediately to the proper antibiotic. I was curable, yet I almost died. I became more self-centered. No more waiting for enough money or the right time or old age. When I want to do something, I do it.

I want to explore this lush earth. My second trip to the Brazilian rain forest was with a World Wildlife Fund guide, who had a Ph.D. in biology, and a collection of natives who carried supplies and cooked. The other six tourists in our group ranged from accountants and architects to environmentalists, all conservation-minded. In a Travelall we drove to an unused army barracks deep in the rain forest. There we made camp, with a barrel of fresh water, thin-mattressed cots, no electricity, and one pit toilet. My bed was next to the pit, and I was the unintentional guidepost as human bodies crawled over me during the night. Overhead rats made scraping sounds on the open rafters, using their toenails to secure footing. Occasionally one became unbalanced and fell on a sleeper. For three days we lived with bugs, sweat, rain, mud, and smothering heat. Then the guides hauled our sodden, stinky bodies to a deluxe hotel. After a shower, we ate the chef's special in clean clothes. Then we laughed about the barracks and agreed they weren't as bad as we expected. Two days later we returned to our jungle camp.

Natives remain healthy in the tropics unvaccinated, but one month before departure, I had to start immunizations against yellow fever, typhoid, cholera, tetanus, and hepatitis. In my suitcase I carried antimalaria and antidiarrhea pills.

On one Amazon River trip, a native guide invited me into his family home. It was a large one-room hut with a dirt floor and a wood fire where a pot was boiling. As my eyes became accustomed to the darkness, I saw small animals scurrying past my feet. I grabbed one and, to my surprise, was staring at a Peruvian guinea pig. The Indian woman smiled and with nods and hand motions offered to boil it for me.

"They are very tasty," the guide explained.

I made it clear I had no appetite for guinea pig.

Closer to home, along the Baja Peninsula, I've seen the breeding grounds of the Pacific gray whale. The whales bear their young in San Ignacio Lagoon, a whale sanctuary, where I floated on a Zodiac raft among huge scarred bodies, close enough to be covered by spray from their blowholes.

I'm at home on land or in the water. In the Amazon rain forests my guide found a pool free from piranhas and crocodiles and pure enough for a cool dip. In Brazil, drinking water was carried in a barrel and tightly rationed. I bathed in a stream, alert for electric eels and stingrays. In Antarctica I even swam in a hot geothermal pool and have the tourist patch to prove it. In Australia I joined a boat crew that allowed me unlimited time to snorkel in the warm currents of the Coral Sea off the Great Barrier Reef. There fish and sea life flourish in such variety that I could go every day of my life and not be bored.

In 1988 I spent four weeks in Australia and discovered the city of Alice Springs, a thousand miles from anywhere, isolated by desert and, in the rainy season, floods. There dust storms and rough roads destroy a Land-Rover's engine in six months. It's cheaper to own an airplane. The residents are tough British sheep ranchers who offer tourists dinner in their homes or buy drinks for them at the friendly all-night bar. Two hundred eighty miles southeast is Ayers Rock, one of the largest monoliths in the world, shoved 1,143 feet above the earth's crust before recorded time. Six miles in circumference, it looks like a surreal mountain glowing red in the afternoon sun.

I don't stay long in large cities. There people are at their worst. Growing populations want everything in their lifetime. They see no need to conserve rich croplands, rain forests, natural resources, wild animals, or even peaceful primitive cultures. If the land is not nurtured, people will exhaust their resources. In the bush, human values are different. There all life is equal. My native guide is my teacher, my companion, my friend. We trust each other with our lives.

I wanted to see Antarctica because I've never been there. I wanted to see the marine mammals, penguins, and wonderful seabirds before they learned to fear humans. I left home thoroughly informed about Antarctica, but until I stood on its surface, I could not begin to imagine its immense size and emptiness.

Except for penguins and marine mammals, all life on the continent is artificial and dependent on supplies from the outside world. No trees, no vegetation, no land animals, no native people. Even airplanes cannot operate in the severe cold of winter. For nine months of winter, Antarctica is a lifeless continent.

The alien humans live in twenty to twenty-five research stations belonging to various countries. Each scientist must be psychologically prepared to adjust to a year of intense solitude.

Strangely enough, among the people in this remote land I saw the same spirit of unselfish cooperation that I saw among tribes in remote Brazilian rain forests. In both places my travel group experienced mechanical failure and received instant skilled help. Severe living conditions seem to break down all barriers, and people truly care for each other, wanting no reward.

I spent ten days of antarctic summer, in January and February, anchored just off the Antarctic Peninsula where a chain of islands offers a hospitable landing. To get to the shore, I boarded a rubber Zodiac raft, a daily adventure. Layered with clothes—

waterproof pants, knee-high boots, heavy parka, hat, mittens, and life preserver—I stood, barely mobile, on the edge of the ship's platform, my arms stretched full-length in front, waiting for two crewmen to lift me from the platform to the raft, rising and falling eight feet below.

The land was rough and rocky, mostly snow and ice with patches of mud and running water occasioned by long hours of daylight and temperatures of thirty to forty degrees Fahrenheit, not counting the wind chill. There was always wind.

I walked among breeding colonies of penguins and seals, and if I didn't rush at them or act erratic, I could get quite close. The penguins were molting and looked ragged instead of sleek, unable to swim because they weren't waterproof. One of my friends sat quietly on a rock. On a rock behind and a little above her, I watched a penguin slowly lean ever further, to get a better view of her. Suddenly he became unbalanced and fell with a *splat* on her back. She ignored him, so he scrambled back on his rock and again began his curious study.

Penguins are the only permanent residents, as all other birds and mammals migrate to warmer land. In winter, when temperatures drop to one hundred degrees Fahrenheit below zero, and wind and blowing snow make existence impossible, the emperor penguin lays her egg. Standing unshielded in the blizzard, she cradles the egg gently on her feet, protecting it with her body warmth until, in a week or two, her mate relieves her. Then she feeds to regain weight. If the egg is not laid in winter, summer is too short for the chick to mature and become self-sufficient.

I saw my first leopard seal, a large carnivore whose eyes are not soft and sweet like those of other seals, as it dives to kill a penguin in the frigid water. I smelled my first minke whale, which has a breath like rotten broccoli and drifted near our raft while we studied each other. I saw floating glaciers five miles across, whose colors glowed blue and shades of pristine white. I loved being there. I must go back.

Perhaps it is my veterinary training that gives me this incredible longing to experience life without civilization, to feel as closely as possible what the wild animal feels. All my contacts with nature enrich me. I carry the heat, the dust, the cold, the wind, the smells, and the wonder of these unaltered experiences in my mind and senses. At home, at work, I remember them from time to time, and they are part of me forever. ■

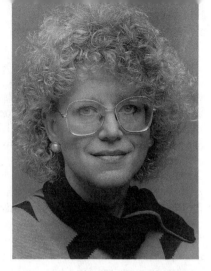

Kathleen Smiler

KATHLEEN SMILER has fashioned success from the polarized elements in her life: a career woman devoted to her four boys; a wife aiming for the top of her profession while coveting a traditional marriage; a veterinarian directing a biomedical laboratory that is a model of humane animal care; a feminist who encourages women to play all roles well. Smiler is a superachiever who has beaten the odds in every category.

Receiving her doctor of veterinary medicine degree from Michigan State University at East Lansing in 1970, Smiler worked two years in a small-animal practice in suburban Detroit, near her hometown. Attracted to veterinary medicine as a science major, Smiler was not completely satisfied dealing with people and pets. In 1972 Smiler became clinical veterinarian and assistant professor of comparative medicine at Wayne State University in Detroit. Directing medical care for the animal research colony, teaching laboratory-animal technicians, and interacting with physicians and Ph.D.'s in human medical research nourished her interest in science.

Her expertise and drive attracted the attention of a Fortune 500

corporation, and she served as its consultant in the design and construction of a modern accredited animal-research facility. In 1976 Smiler was hired by the corporation as senior staff veterinarian and was given responsibility for all of its animal-use programs. "Only a person with compassion for animals belongs in a research laboratory," Smiler says. "No one is better trained to understand animal health and prevent animal distress than a veterinarian."

In 1982 Smiler realized that the impact of the increasing number of women in the veterinary profession could not be ignored, and she joined the Association for Women Veterinarians. Elected president of the organization in 1986, she became an effective spokesperson for women's issues. As a member emeritus of the Michigan State College of Veterinary Medicine alumni council, Smiler has counseled many technicians and veterinary students on career opportunities and has led discussions concerning problems faced by these young career women.

A laboratory-animal veterinarian without benefit of formal residency training, Smiler used enormous self-drive to achieve the ultimate goal of her career in July 1989, when she was accepted into the American College of Laboratory Animal Medicine. Now she sits with the best and brightest of her profession.

In laboratory-animal medicine and as a feminist leader Smiler applies the same workable philosophy: "I flex. I try to make everything fun. It's not that I don't do my best, but if it doesn't work out, I laugh and come back at it from another angle."

■

I could be the modern American dream. I graduated from high school, earned a doctor of veterinary medicine degree, built a stable marriage, mothered four boys, and found pleasure in a career that suits me perfectly. My parents are growing older with grandchildren they adore and a daughter who can help them savor their retirement.

My childhood wasn't particularly marked for success. My mother operated a boarding kennel and became a well-known breeder of parti-colored cocker spaniels. My dad operated a Mobil Oil gas station until the kennel earned a profit. Then he became the kennel's business manager so Mom could concentrate on her cockers. He enlarged the forty-dog building into a two-hundred-dog enterprise, and he and Mom were bound to their business for forty years.

I was an only child who cleaned and raked dog runs after school and during the summer worked fourteen-hour days in the kennel. On weekends I lugged our dogs to dog shows. Well supervised by my parents, I mingled mostly with their friends and other people at the dog shows. I grew up acting like a little adult with glasses, very tolerant, very mature. As a teenager, I was still sheltered. A year younger than my classmates, I didn't date. When I was sixteen, my parents first allowed me to ride in a car with a girlfriend.

All my childhood contacts with animals were strictly business and hard work. My parents lived on seven acres in the suburbs, where, in addition to the kennel, they maintained a goat herd. I asked for a horse, but instead I was kept busy milking and feeding goats and showing my dog in junior showmanship and obedience.

193

At the dog shows, I became good friends with Leonard Smiler, who was always joking with breeders and helping us carry in our dog crates. He was a businessman who developed and sold folding wire dog crates, and all the dog people loved him, including my parents. At that time I barely noticed his quiet son, Joel, who was my age. Our parents never imagined that the two of us would meet in veterinary school and, worse yet, marry. My family was Polish Catholic, and Joel's was Jewish.

A great deal of my youth was also spent waiting in Dr. Fred Gasow's veterinary hospital while he treated my mother's cockers. I admired Dr. Gasow but was not drawn strongly to veterinary medicine.

I was one of two girls in the science and engineering curriculum at our high school and associated with a small group of "brains." I was the favorite pupil of my science teachers, who were emboldened by my high test scores. I was bright, and that was all. I planned to become a pure scientist.

As a National Merit Scholarship semifinalist, I was courted by several universities. I chose Michigan State in East Lansing because it had a veterinary college. Deeply buried was the nagging notion that I might become a veterinarian. I enrolled in interdisciplinary biological science and lived on the opposite end of the campus from the preveterinary students.

One day I was walking past the basic science building and heard dogs barking. A rush of familiarity and fondness for our family dogs surfaced so suddenly that I knew I had to be a veterinarian. The next day, I changed my major.

Some students are attracted to veterinary medicine as animal lovers; others, by the lure of medicine. I came as a scientist who thought the study of animal disease would give me some sense of order and well-being.

The broad array of science courses seemed to work for me. Both parents approved my career choice. Father adored me and felt I was no more limited than a son. Father had studied metallurgy in college but did not graduate, and he never forgot this disappointment.

Mother had actually been in preveterinary medicine at Michigan State a short time during the war. In those days it was so difficult for a woman to gain acceptance into the veterinary college that she did not apply. Instead she married my father. Mother always encouraged my career, and at times I suspected she envied me.

Michigan State allowed 20 percent women in the freshman class, a higher percentage than any other veterinary college. Male and female students mixed into one fun-loving group. Even the faculty was accustomed to women. The only small problem I remember was an old-time clinician who believed students should strip to the waist to clean a cow [remove the rotting placenta from the uterus].

I was one of nine women in a class of fifty, and forty graduated, including all nine women. In the past, women may have had to sacrifice some femininity to be veterinarians, but my female classmates were attractive, polished, and datable. We wore skirts to class, and the men wore shirts and ties. My intelligence was admired, and always mature, I became a leader of sorts. During those years my self-confidence bloomed.

As a freshman veterinary student, I applied at Giltner Hall, the basic science building, for a job cleaning kennels. I was told that Dr. Ray Johnston was in charge of dogs for the physiology lab. I found his room and knocked on the closed door. An aging man in a white lab coat frowned at me.

"I came to apply for kennel work," I said.

"We don't hire girls," he grumbled.

"Wait!" I wedged my body in the door. "There's nothing I haven't done."

"What do you mean?" he asked.

"I've worked in a dog kennel all my life. I can breed bitches, run stud dogs, whelp puppies. I can do anything."

"Come in," he said.

Thus began my apprenticeship with Dr. Johnston, a veterinarian with a Ph.D. in physiology. He stood by my side all four years of veterinary school and spurred my resolve to be a veterinarian.

Dr. Johnston was developing a colony of special inbred labrador retrievers for a scientist who was studying the effects of renal hypertension. I was placed in charge of his initial stock, three pregnant AKC bitches and a stud dog. During my four years in veterinary school, I bred bitches, whelped puppies, put bitches out on loan, and brought them back to breed to our stud dogs. This work gave me considerably more exposure to medical research than my classmates received.

In those days everyone wanted to be a veterinarian. Six or more applicants applied for every opening in veterinary school. In the battle to enter, a woman's grade point had to be higher (2.98) than a man's (2.5). This selected for female superachievers who were less likely to drop out than the men. After graduation, most of these women continued in successful careers. Today enrollment is dropping, and entrance requirements are more equal for both sexes. Without intense competition, a more average student is accepted, different from our group in personality, goals, priorities, and background.

I wasn't aware of sex discrimination until I graduated. Then it hit me like a cold shower. I wrote thirty-five letters of application to small-animal hospitals in the Detroit area. Two veterinarians offered an interview. One of the two was only curious to see what I looked like. My fiancé was already employed at a practice in the same area, and this seemed to make me less desirable. Finally my father talked to Dr. Gasow, who had hired me summers when I was a student. "I just put Kathleen through eight years of veterinary school, and nobody wants to hire her," my dad complained.

Dr. Gasow already had eight associates, but he graciously hired me. His small-animal practice was very progressive, with high-tech veterinarians who specialized in surgery, dermatology, and ophthalmology. Being new, I handled clients in the exam rooms and gained general experience. All those years in my mother's dog business soon made me popular with dog breeders, and if Dr. Gasow was gone, they asked for me. Other than that, I didn't distinguish myself. I refused to come in for night emergencies when I learned that the night kennelman might try to hug and kiss me if I came in alone. I was newly married and lived farther from the practice than the other associates. I thought it was fair to substitute twelve-hour days and weekends for night call.

Dr. Gasow was from the old school of veterinarians who were willing to work day and night. Without appointments, twelve people might walk in at 8:30 P.M. for radiographs, and he would accommodate all of them. In two years I had enough experience to convince me that I was competent.

The fall after I graduated, I married Joel. After becoming acquainted during my dog-show days, we had rediscovered each other when we worked the same summer for Dr. Gasow. Later we both attended Michigan State University College of Veterinary Medicine and dated off and on during those four years. Joel graduated from Michigan State six months ahead of me. He wanted his own practice, so we found separate jobs and saved our money. When Joel bought land in Rochester, a Detroit suburb near Dr.

Gasow, I left Dr. Gasow's practice to avoid any conflict of interest. After Joel's hospital was built, we planned to practice together.

In the sixties the Federal Animal Welfare Act was revised and strengthened, so that all medical facilities using animals for research had to be supervised by a veterinarian. The animals were the winners. Veterinarians, well trained in animal health, had great empathy for animal suffering and insured the use of anesthetics to relieve distress.

Wayne State, in Detroit, was revitalizing its entire division of laboratory animal resources and hired a veterinarian from California, well known in the field, as its new director. He advertised for clinicians to care for the animal colony, and I applied. This time I was quickly hired. I was qualified, but even more important, I was a woman needed to meet affirmative action goals.

My title was clinical veterinarian and assistant professor of comparative medicine. I was responsible for the health of all research animals at Wayne State and was a consultant to the university's satellite clinics. I taught laboratory-animal technicians and administered the hospital pharmacy, surgery, and stores. Unlike practice, where I never felt necessary, almost at once I was a viable part of the medical community. Working mostly with dogs and a small number of random species, I improved their health, set up quarantine for new animals, planned preventive medicine, and of course treated the sick. This used my formal education, what I'd learned as a child in my mother's kennel, and what I'd learned working for Dr. Johnston in the basic science building at Michigan State.

I belonged in laboratory-animal medicine and decided not to return to practice. It was just as well. I worked briefly in my husband's animal hospital, and we drove each other crazy. We both wanted to be boss.

A Fortune 500 corporation in Detroit, in the planning stage for a modern research laboratory, contacted me at Wayne State. I was asked to consult with its architects and engineers. What a learning experience! Funds at universities are always limited, and by comparison, this corporation seemed unconcerned with cost. It encouraged me to conceive a facility better equipped than any in the state. To accomplish this, I sought information and advice from the staff at the University of Michigan Medical School. At that time the school was teaching a postdoctoral course in laboratory-animal medicine.

The new research facility was completed in 1976. The

corporation employed me as senior staff veterinarian with complete responsibility for all the animal-use programs. I compared this position with my four years at Wayne State and immediately realized that research in an industrial laboratory had a narrow focus on company problems. If industry lacked variety, it didn't lack financing and efficient management. I was able to organize a laboratory that functioned very close to perfection. I think it was a smart trade-off. Our private facility is accredited by the American Association for Accreditation of Laboratory Animal Care. This association continues to inspect our laboratory and rarely suggests improvements. After fourteen years we're still an exemplary model. Professors at the University of Michigan tour our facility with their postgraduate laboratory-animal residents.

Most of the research at our facility is conducted by Ph.D.'s in toxicology, biochemistry, and engineering. These scientists explore a concept in much greater depth than a veterinarian does. They challenge me, and I love the intellectual stimulation.

Our research species are rats bred for this purpose. While these animals are in research, I ensure humane care, the least discomfort, and all their daily needs. Only healthy rats provide reliable data. Every animal we use makes a significant contribution to human health and safety.

I apply the herd health theory in our rodent colony and quickly remove sick individuals. They are sent to pathology for diagnosis, and I use this information to save the colony from infection.

Scientists with specialty degrees conceive our research projects, but I collaborate to ensure proper handling of the animal. I am sensitive to the value of this animal's life and, whenever possible, devise alternatives to its use.

Most people in the United States believe that animals should be used in medical research. Still there are times I don't like to admit I'm a laboratory-animal veterinarian. I don't think the public is aware of the extensive regulations that protect laboratory animals. Many people in my field, such as veterinarians, veterinary technicians, and laboratory directors, devote their lives to improving conditions for research animals. Being a mother, I'm especially moved when I know that animals have helped children. To me this is a noble calling.

With so many philosophical levels, I sometimes wonder how people can be so certain they have the one right answer. Animal-rights people believe that beef cows should not be slaughtered, dairy cows should not be milked, and no animal should be subjected to research. I can't support this view.

On the other hand, I am violently opposed to hunting. No one has the right to march through the woods, shooting animals for the sheer joy of killing. It's a barbaric game. Hunting-license fees feed the deer and inflate the herd to save large numbers for the public to kill. If the deer population really needs to be culled, the state should hire professional sharpshooters and stop the public from shooting the animals and each other.

When my uncle was alive, he hunted moose every year in northern Ontario. Sometimes he would wound a moose, track the dying beast for several days, then slaughter it for the meat and maybe a moose head. What purpose does that serve?

I teach my children reverence for animals. They don't have guns. I respect God's covenant to use animals wisely and well. I believe that includes using animals for food and medical research.

As a veterinarian, I'm aware of the importance of pets. Sometimes I think we carry this importance too far when we teach veterinary students to perform open-heart surgery on an aging poodle. How can taxpayers justify enormous sums of money to improve the medical care of dogs and cats when that money could be used to save people? Our finances are limited. Maybe we should send veterinary students to Africa for a year to save starving children. Aren't our priorities nonsensical? How important is the life of one dog? I question these things, but I don't pretend to have the answers.

My foremost goal was to become a diplomate of the American College of Laboratory Animal Medicine. The requirements for membership established by the credentials committee were very demanding. I had to publish results from my own research in a refereed science journal and pass an all-day comprehensive examination. I invested three years of preparation. The time I wanted to spend with my family was used for study. While I was dictating self-study tapes about nematodes in spider monkeys, my five-year-old would fall asleep beside me waiting for a bedtime story.

Six months before the exam, Joel and I leased my parents' kennel business. I wanted the kennel, with its memories, to stay in our family, but this was not the best time to take over the business.

Three months before the exam, I had spinal surgery to correct two subluxated cervical vertebrae and came home with a neck brace. Through all this, I met regularly with three other women veterinarians. Like me, they were trying to become certified without the luxury of a postgraduate residency. All of us worked full-time in high-level positions while we studied. Our combined expertise in laboratory-animal medicine, as my boys would say, was awesome.

With the support of my family and these close friends, I passed the examination. In July 1989 I joined the elite in the American College of Laboratory Animal Medicine. I was accepted by board members whom I'd admired for years. The thrill was almost beyond expression.

Now I am anxious to get on with my life and career. I'd like to follow my interest in new anesthetics and analgesics and find better ways to make animals comfortable and monitor their vital functions under anesthesia.

Just as important, I want to spend time with my husband and four boys, ages six to fifteen. My first son was born after five years of marriage. With dual veterinary careers, my husband and I have the resources to hire good care for our children. We found a wonderful young woman who runs our family during the week. When I leave for work, she's there to prepare meals for my boys, get them ready for school, drive them to appointments, and mother them when they need it. I come home to a clean house, my dinner and Joel's ready for the microwave, and boys who have eaten and are busy with homework or other projects. When I was home recovering from neck surgery, my youngest sometimes wondered if I or his temporary mom was in charge. With this kind of support, my children are raised in their home with their neighborhood friends. If I were home all the time, harried and fussing, I wouldn't do any better than I do now.

Joel is a wonderful father. His veterinary hospital is nearby, and he is able to spend considerable time with the children. Some weekends we take nine boys—ours and some of their friends—on trips. Family vacations are our relaxed time together. When we owned a travel trailer, we spent several weeks each summer exploring national parks. At Christmas we head west. Sometimes we stay at a dude ranch and ride horses; other times, at a mountain resort in New Mexico, where we ski. Our boys have seen almost every state, including Hawaii. If Joel and I worked in the same practice, we would never have all this time together.

I don't think Joel expected me to be such an overachiever. He built up his business so I could stay home. But I must use my education. We handle my competitive nature with a sense of humor. Our careers are so different that we stay interested in each other.

In Joel's peer group I'm the oddball. Practitioners think I work in research because I don't have the stamina to succeed in practice. Joel is the successful businessperson. My high salary and benefits don't threaten Joel's ego or self-respect. Among our old friends, practice is the real world and lab-animal medicine is monotony. For romance, Joel and I relax, without children, at a heartworm symposium or my laboratory-animal convention. We soak up education during the day and have fun with our colleagues at night.

As the number of women increased rapidly in veterinary medicine, I realized that someone had to work out intelligent solutions to their concerns. I joined the Association for Women Veterinarians (AWV) to help integrate women into the profession. This organization was established in 1947 to meet the needs of a small number of isolated women. As membership increased, AWV changed its focus to address important issues overlooked by other veterinary organizations. The association has an overworked core of volunteers who somehow manage to turn out the same yearly accomplishments: a seminar at the American Veterinary Medical Association convention, scholarships to veterinary students, an award to the Outstanding Woman Veterinarian of the Year, and the Distinguished Service Award for an individual, male or female, who helps the cause of women. Women veterinarians need their own peer group while they gain the confidence and experience to succeed with men. Women's issues are touchy, but our Association for Women Veterinarians can discuss these issues freely and not be accused of discrimination.

I joined AWV as central director in 1982, became president-elect in 1984, president in 1986, and treasurer in 1988. As president, I had to find an interesting subject for our yearly seminar. The two topics that drew the most enthusiasm were health hazards in veterinary practice, including protection for the unborn, and maternity benefits. We formed the maternity and women's health issues committee, chaired by Dr. Carol Hogfoss Rubin, who was well qualified to find speakers and gather pertinent, meaningful information. By keeping our issues relevant to women, we don't compete with other associations. The officers stimulate networking and find successful female role models for new graduates.

During my two years as president, I learned to be less outrageous in my views, to temper my statements with "This is my opinion." My beliefs mellowed a bit, but I still have a great deal of empathy for young couples with their first baby. Society must make temporary allowances for professional women. This two-track model, in which women with children should climb a separate career ladder, is ridiculous. Only the first baby is hard. If employers are tolerant and let the new mother get things under control, she'll come back to work and work as hard as ever. Too many practices assume pregnant women aren't coming back. One workable solution is for the new mother to return to work gradually on a part-time basis. She could relieve her employer three or four hours a day during heavy work periods. When mothers try to work a full eight-to-ten-hour day before the baby is twelve weeks old, they only prolong their exhaustion. If intelligent, creative career women are penalized for having children, what kind of mothers will we have?

My employers were very tolerant of my four pregnancies. I worked at the university when my first child was born. The first month, I stayed at home and felt so incompetent that I wanted to return my son and get my money back. After four months at home, I couldn't wait to get back to work. Then at work I felt guilty. My mother-in-law assumed I would resign. Everybody was watching Brian, my cute little red-haired son, to see if he would be ruined. Remember that in the seventies most mothers didn't work, pediatricians didn't make evening appointments, and child care was not a national issue. Joel and I couldn't yet afford a baby-sitter, so Brian went to work with his father.

As soon as we hired a full-time housekeeper, I continued having children. I loved being pregnant. I was so blasé about my due date that one time I attended a Big Ten football game and another time traveled to Seattle, Washington, on business, shortly before delivery. I adore babies, but four boys are enough. Now they are all at the age when our family can enjoy outdoor activities together.

With my second son, the corporation allowed a two-month leave. With my third son, I returned part-time in a few weeks. I met all my responsibilities while I gradually increased to full-time hours. When my last son, Peter, was born, I returned to work in six days. I called it a one-week disability leave.

Women veterinary students enjoy the majority status in veterinary college, but when they look for work, they find a male-dominated profession. Through my work on the Alumni council at Michigan State, I've helped female students decide what to say during an interview. We discuss how they should present their personal life and how they should negotiate for benefits, especially maternity. Small-town employers like to ask personal questions about religion, family life, social habits, and significant others. By law, they cannot ask these questions or hold the answers against a student. Times are changing.

With two dominant careers, Joel and I together solve the problems of rearing a family. We compromise frequently. Fortunately, my personality absorbs catastrophes. It's a gift I have. I suffer two days at most, then bounce back with another solution. At work, surrounded by sensitive male intellectuals, I avoid ultimatums. I never say "No!" or "I won't do this." This has even saved arguments with my husband and in-laws. For example, my husband does our long-range planning. He makes daily, weekly, and monthly lists and crosses off his accomplishments. I facilitate short-term plans and manage last-minute crises. Sometimes I have many plans in action at one time. Our opposite traits are effective.

If I wrote an advice column, I'd tell young women never to marry on a whim. Look at the man they intend to marry, and try to picture what he'll be like in twenty years. Carefully consider the values of his family. Do you share their goals? Joel and I have been so united these twenty years that we've managed to build a life we both want. I have been able to balance both my career and my family. This life-style is not for every professional woman, but for those who want to try, all they need is a tremendous reserve of energy. If women continue to combine children and career, veterinarians will be forced to find solutions agreeable to both men and women. ■

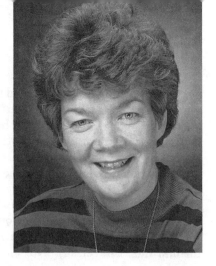

Barbara Soderstrom

WHEN Barbara Soderstrom earned her doctor of veterinary medicine degree from the University of Illinois College of Veterinary Medicine in 1964, she envisioned an exciting career in small-animal medicine. That did not seem too much to expect. After all, from the age of eleven, all through high school and college, even while working summers at a small-animal hospital, Barbara had dreamed of becoming a veterinarian. Her highest grades in veterinary school were in the clinics where she was able to work with the animals. Why then, after six years in small-animal practice, did she long to do something different?

This longing made Barbara and her husband, Leonard, decide to change their life-style. At a time when their friends wanted secure jobs with high pay, Barbara and Len quit work, left the frenzy of their Chicago suburb, and sought a peaceful place where they could relax and find jobs they enjoyed.

The Soderstroms discovered utopia in the warm, fragrant woods of North Carolina. There Barbara accepted a job with the U.S. Department of Agriculture's Food Safety and Inspection Service (FSIS). To her surprise, she found fulfillment as a poultry inspector.

Barbara Soderstrom joined the inspection service when the poultry industry was expanding rapidly. Americans, long known as beef eaters, were switching to chicken and turkey. Her veterinary credentials involved her in a fascinating journey: first as an inspector in charge of three turkey-processing plants in North Carolina, then as a teacher on the training staff at the FSIS training center in Fort Worth, Texas, and finally to her present position with training headquarters in Denton, Texas.

Writing, editing, speaking, teaching, and constantly gathering and updating information related to the poultry industry, Soderstrom is a one-person information center. Her publications and videos provide up-to-date instruction for veterinary poultry inspectors and are also an important reference for veterinary colleges and private poultry producers.

Once a year Soderstrom teaches a one-week course, which she designed, on the U.S. poultry inspection system. Her pupils are foreign veterinarians and sanitarians with inspection respon-sibilities in their own countries. Over the years, more than fifteen foreign countries have participated.

"After all the blood, sweat, and tears of veterinary college, I'm amazed to find the poultry industry so fascinating," Soderstrom says. "This job has helped me learn a lot about myself, about the world I live in, how big business and government operate, and how I can affect these institutions. As a new graduate, I really didn't know myself. Now I do. Working at what I like, I've matured."

■

My dad, a Chicago police officer, impounded a collie at our neighborhood animal hospital because the dog bit someone. At the end of the ten-day observation period, the owners no longer wanted their dog. The veterinarian, Dr. Grant Meisner, talked my parents into adopting it. The collie was young and healthy and didn't deserve to be euthanized.

Mother really didn't want a dog, but there was a serial murderer at large in our neighborhood, and with Dad working nights, she agreed to take the collie for protection. Lance became part of our family. My job was to care for Lance, and because he wasn't as healthy as we thought, that included numerous trips to the veterinarian. In a short time I became good friends with Dr. Meisner.

Dr. Meisner and Lance, my first dog, inspired me to be a veterinarian. At age eleven, I made a firm commitment and never considered any other career. In a way it was strange. Looking back, I don't remember being a fanatic pet-keeper. I liked animals, but my interests were well balanced. I was a typical teenage girl with very feminine ideas who also played basketball and other sports with the boys.

Both my parents came from families who lost their wealth during the Depression. They didn't own a car until I was eleven, and they bought their first house, on Chicago's north side, when I was fifteen. My mother worked part-time at first and later full-time as a claims clerk for a railroad. Dad was proud of her. He used to brag that her job paid more than his.

Neither of my parents went to college, but both preached that a good education bestowed financial independence and the opportunity to find rewarding work. As a Chicago police officer in the 1940s and 1950s, Dad saw women who were trapped in terrible domestic relationships because they were totally dependent on their husbands. Naturally, my parents wanted me to be independent, and they encouraged my interest in veterinary medicine.

In preveterinary medicine at De Paul University in Chicago, I had a mandatory (I didn't think I needed any counseling) meeting with my guidance counselor. A well-respected priest on the faculty, he asked, "Why do you want to be a veterinarian? All those years of education and study, and you're only going to get married." I remember being a little bit irritated but not in the least discouraged.

At the start of my sophomore year I couldn't get a required course at De Paul, so I transferred to the Chicago campus of the University of Illinois, at Navy Pier near downtown Chicago. My preveterinary work was complete in two years, and the University of Illinois accepted me into its College of Veterinary Medicine.

I was one of two women in a class of thirty-nine. A few of the men appeared to think that we didn't belong. At the time, I was more or less oblivious to these attitudes. I knew I was perfectly feminine and had no doubt about my goals. My self-confidence probably made me less sensitive to biased comments.

Early in my freshman year of veterinary school, I met a young teacher from a nearby town. It turned out that he was friends with several of my classmates, and at times the entire class seemed to conduct my romance. By Christmas my boyfriend was suggesting marriage. I should quit school, he thought, and depend on him. Because I had no interest in marriage or dropping out of school, our relationship began to fade. The deathblow occurred when I suggested we visit the veterinary anatomy room. We were alone with embalmed horses and cows suspended from the ceiling by meat hooks. I put on an animated show of muscles and livers and stomachs and eyeballs while he turned green. Shortly after, he lost all interest in me.

As a four-year member of the veterinary fraternity, Omega Tau Sigma (OTS), I enjoyed close camaraderie with my classmates, even serving as fraternity secretary and historian. I have faint memories of a wild weekend in Guelph, Ontario, at the international convention of OTS. I may have been the only female fraternity member there. Other fraternity chapters were not as liberal as the one at Illinois.

After I received my doctor of veterinary medicine degree in 1964, I worked in a small-animal practice in Chicago for Dr. Leonard Tovell, a close friend of Dr. Meisner's. It wasn't long before I felt the pressure of practice. I seemed to be worried about something most of the time. Had I made the correct diagnosis? Was the pet improving? Had my treatment enhanced recovery? Could I have done more? After a long day dealing with emotional pet owners, I would flinch when the phone rang at my home. Too often it was an emergency. It seemed my life was not my own, especially when Dr. Tovell was away and I was in charge.

After two long years of practice, I tried relief work. I practiced three days a week, one with Dr. Tovell and the remaining days at two other hospitals. Occasionally I'd work a full week or two when a veterinarian was vacationing. I took no night calls, saw relatively few clients, and concentrated on treating hospital patients and performing surgery. My hours had improved, but I never looked forward to work and was relieved when the day ended.

While I struggled to fit into practice, I married my husband, Leonard. We met while I was still in veterinary college. My parents and Len's aunt and uncle were close friends. I stayed with Len's aunt and uncle in Chicago over Easter vacation. The aunt was anxious for me to meet Len and arranged a blind date. At first sight, Len and I liked each other. After three fun-filled evenings of nonstop conversation, I returned to my third year in the veterinary college and convinced myself that Len and I had nothing in common. I was pursuing a veterinary career, and he was a lithographer with no college education—not the right ingredients for a serious relationship.

When I began practice in Chicago, Len was living there also. We started dating, and although we dated others, our strong attraction for each other remained. After four years of quiet waiting, my mother, who was fond of Len, gave me some advice. "That man loves you and wants to marry you," she said. "If you don't feel the same about him, tell him. Stop stringing him along." I realized then that I cared very much for him, and two months later we were married.

From the beginning, I told Len I didn't want children. My parents never pushed marriage or motherhood, even though I had several girlfriends who were married in their early twenties. All immediately had children. Pregnancy and childbirth looked unappealing. Their children needed so much attention that these young women had no time or opportunity for other interests. This wasn't for me. Leonard said the decision was mine because my life would be most affected. With Leonard in agreement, we remained childless by choice. Eventually our family and friends accepted our attitude and stopped offering advice and opinions.

Len and I lived in an apartment in a crowded suburb of Chicago. I was working three days a week, and he was in management at a large printing company. We were following carefully chosen careers. We had money and wonderful friends. Still, we felt dissatisfied. It wasn't easy, but we had to admit we didn't like our jobs. Once we faced the cause of our unhappiness, we made careful plans to alter our life-style.

For one year we kept a tight budget, then quit our jobs and sold almost everything we owned. A new car, equipped for towing, and an eight-by-twenty-four-foot travel trailer became our home. I was thirty and Len was thirty-four when we began our venture to find a place with less population, less traffic, less hassle, and warmer winters than Chicago. Location was our first priority; then we would look for jobs. We were excited and scared. Well-meaning friends told us we were nuts.

We stayed six weeks in Florida and found crowds, traffic, pollution, and palm trees. We pushed on, up the East Coast, heading for a family reunion in Missouri, and passed through North Carolina. Almost immediately we liked that state, the flowering dogwood, the rolling green hills, the smiling people, and the comfortable climate. Still, we stuck to our travel plans and took time to explore Oregon, Washington, California, and the states in between. After ten months we returned to North Carolina, eager to settle there.

Near Charlotte we rented a space in a trailer park for twenty-five dollars a month. Our travel money was gone, but Len stirred up two job offers the first day and was working by the second. With his Chicago experience, the Charlotte printing companies wanted him to manage, but he refused those headaches and started as a lithographer.

Looking for an alternative to practice, I thumbed through the *Journal of the American Veterinary Medical Association.* The U.S. Department of Agriculture was advertising for veterinarians and listed a job in a poultry plant in, of all places, Charlotte. A few months later I was hired and was on my way to Fort Worth, Texas, for nine weeks of intensive training in inspection. I returned to Charlotte as the supervisor of the poultry plant.

A year later I was transferred as the inspector in charge of three turkey-processing plants in Monroe, North Carolina, thirty miles to the south. This move brought me closer to Waxhaw, where we were building a house on fourteen acres of woods enlivened by a stream.

The public thinks government work is easy. It's not. I drove a hundred miles a day, five days a week. Among the three plants, I often put in ten-hour days supervising as many as fifteen food inspectors and another veterinarian. In addition I'd drive to South Carolina to make the final disposition on an abnormal carcass detected by a solitary inspector at a small meat processing plant.

Food inspectors in a poultry plant are stationed on the postmortem line, inspecting each carcass for signs of disease or contamination. They have the authority either to condemn the abnormal carcass or to retain the carcass for the veterinarian's judgment. As the veterinary supervisor, I was responsible for the inspectors' decisions, so I watched postmortem, where disease is most evident, carefully. Every process in the plant was checked by food inspectors to be sure that only wholesome products reached the market. These inspectors discussed simple problems with company supervisors and notified me only about major issues. Some days there seemed to be a crisis every hour.

One long, hot summer a drought lowered the water level in the municipal reservoir, and a stirring effect occurred. Bottom sludge, which contained many minerals from the soil, got into the water supply. These minerals combined with chlorine and other substances to produce a black compound that unfortunately adhered to the poultry carcass. Because water is used in every operation in a slaughter plant, most turkeys looked like they had been sprayed with motor oil. The material was nontoxic, but the turkeys were legally adulterated. I stopped production and retained the black carcasses. Production stopped so often that summer that the owners threatened to sue me. I stood my ground, and my supervisors gave me total support. Over and over I explained my actions to city officials and plant managers. The inspectors developed acute eyestrain watching for foreign matter on turkeys. Everyone was overjoyed when rain finally came and solved the problem.

My legal authority was clearly spelled out in the federal poultry inspection regulations and manuals, but I still had to apply common sense and judgment. When plant management tried to do a good job, I tried to help rather than hinder by overzealous use of my authority. The intent of federal inspection was not to make life miserable for business by stringent enforcement, but rather to encourage business to comply with good manufacturing practices that gave consumers a quality product. On the other hand, I had little sympathy for dishonest or sloppy operations and made rules stick tightly until management improved to get me out of its hair.

I used this philosophy in the plants and now convey it in my training programs.

The poultry industry is extremely competitive but sees an advantage to government inspection as long as the rules are enforced uniformly. Careful inspection discourages processors who would cut corners to gain advantage over competitors.

Although federal inspection of red meat (beef, pork, and lamb) has existed since 1906, poultry inspection wasn't enforced until 1958. Before World War II the poultry industry was mostly a sideline of egg production. Male chicks were raised to market size, and spent hens, which no longer were productive egg layers, were sold to small local slaughter plants. During World War II a fast-growing alternate source of meat protein was needed for the consumer because most of the red meat was shipped to the armed forces. Raising chickens for meat suddenly became profitable. The government funded research in genetics, disease control, and nutrition, and poultry production developed rapidly into a major U.S. industry.

Relative to red meat, poultry is quite perishable. Before proper refrigeration was developed, birds were shipped live to plants located near major markets. There were many losses due to death and disease in transit. Now birds are slaughtered close to where they are raised, and the meat quickly refrigerated or frozen for shipping great distances.

I am fascinated by the efficiency and new ideas of the poultry industry. It rivals science fiction when a newly hatched turkey poult, weighing only a few ounces, will grow to twenty pounds in only four months. Even baby chicks attain a market weight of four pounds in about six weeks.

Bred to resist disease, today's birds are plumped with growth stimulants and precise nutrition. Disease is controlled with regular vaccination and low-level antibiotics. Flocks are watched closely, and at the first sign of sickness, samples are taken to a laboratory for quick diagnosis to keep bird losses to a minimum.

Although there are small poultry farms that still cater to the whim of the consumer, most poultry production is big business. Slaughter plants easily process a quarter million birds in a day. Large companies own every phase of the operation, from breeding stock to feed mill to slaughter plant. They usually pay private farmers to build poultry houses and act as caretakers for the birds. This arrangement eliminates the intermediate agent and keeps the cost of poultry products low.

Eventually all birds raised for food come to the slaughter plant, where government inspectors ensure the public a safe wholesome food. Regularly I am asked if I eat chicken or turkey. The assumption is that insiders wouldn't. Well, I am on the inside and eat poultry, a lot of it.

The day after "60 Minutes" presented its exposé of the poultry industry, I was the featured speaker at a women's club. Poultry inspectors were suddenly not popular. Many of those educated affluent women had just purged their home of poultry to save their family from *Salmonella* poisoning or some other horrible disease. I made a valiant effort to correct the misinformation broadcast by the boob tube.

The longer I'm involved with inspection, the more frustrated I become with improper food handling in homes and restaurants that can cause food-borne illness. Poultry should be adequately cooked, quickly refrigerated, and prepared on nonabsorbing kitchen surfaces. Most important, these surfaces should be washed with hot soapy water.

I derive a great deal of satisfaction from a neat, clean environment. Inspecting poultry plants seemed to suit this part of my personality and even reward it with a paycheck and the pleasure of protecting people's health.

After a few years my work in the poultry plants seemed under control, and I took on the additional job of Federal Women's Program manager for the southeastern region. This voluntary part-time duty made me a member of an Equal Employment Opportunity (EEO) committee. I became a bridge between women employees in the agency and upper management. If women felt they were victims of discrimination, harassment, or some other injustice, I showed them how EEO rules could help. I took courses in equal employment laws, civil rights, public speaking, and cultural awareness and attended conventions aimed at helping women in government.

Slaughter plants, especially those for red meat, are a traditional male environment. Until recent years there were few female employees and even fewer female inspectors. Change began about fifteen years ago and was not always welcome. Female inspectors often met with hostility, even overt harassment, from company employees and male inspectors. Food Safety Inspection Service managers tried to eliminate this behavior. They encouraged me as regional Federal Women's Program manager to improve attitudes toward women.

I put together a somewhat provocative speech on sexual harassment and spoke at various agency meetings throughout the Southeast. I warned the audience that we were discussing a highly emotional subject. Experts list many reasons why problems occur between the genders, and I discussed the most likely. I did not expect people to accept or agree with everything I said, but to consider it as food for thought.

On one occasion I was about to speak to forty male veterinarians when I recognized a man in the audience who had given me trouble in the past. During my speech I sensed his growing agitation. As I concluded, he leaped to his feet to speak his mind and, among other things, label me a lesbian, an atheist, and possibly a Communist. The rest of the audience squirmed in discomfort. Then he ran out of words and sat down. I gave him what I hoped was a sincere-looking smile and thanked him for his remarks.

During a break my colleagues apologized for this man's abusive remarks and congratulated me for maintaining control of the situation and myself. Ten years later I still met men who were impressed by that session. That irate man did more to boost my career and sensitize men to the nastiness of discrimination than anything I could have planned.

Living in a rural area has many charms, but some things that city folks take for granted are nonexistent, such as paid fire and ambulance service. We lived five miles out of town and often had a long wait for the ambulance. Because I was the only person in our neighborhood with medical training, an injured neighbor sometimes asked for my help. Worried about the consequences of a mistake, I with my husband joined the volunteer emergency medical team in Waxhaw. We were trained to be certified emergency medical technicians (EMTs).

We attended three-hour classes two nights a week for three months. We worked in the emergency room of a hospital for two weekends and passed a written and practical examination that lasted eight hours. My veterinary education did not make the course easy. I haven't studied that hard since veterinary school, and my nonmedical classmates had even more difficulty.

Most of us received our official credentials. Then we worried about our first ambulance call. Would we stay calm, perform properly, and not get sick at some horrible sight? Len and I soon found out. A drunk driver with a passenger in the front seat had a head-on collision with a truck close to our house. Neither victim had been wearing a seat belt, and when we arrived, we found hysterical people covered with blood and pulverized glass. Our new skills gave us the confidence to help these people. We came away knowing we had gained more from our training than we had put into it. Len and I have great admiration for EMTs and volunteer fire fighters.

My participation in ancillary government activities earned friends for me in management. When the Food Safety Inspection Service training center in Fort Worth needed an instructor, the head of the training division wanted me to join his team. After ten years in the slaughter plants, it was exciting to return to the education center and train new inspectors.

I left for Texas before our house in North Carolina sold, so Len stayed until a buyer was found. I rented an apartment in Denton, a few miles from Fort Worth. For a year and a half, our marriage was long-distance. I loved my new job, but I missed Len. The real estate market was terrible everywhere, and in North Carolina, mortgage interest rates were more than 17 percent. Finally I took a nine-month leave of absence and returned home.

Len and I tried to think out a solution. While we juggled ideas, Len received a call from the Graphic Arts Foundation, asking him to join its staff of consultants. Backed by the foundation's authority and prestige, Len would travel across the United States and into foreign countries, solving problems for the printing industry. "Of course," the caller explained, "he must be based in Texas."

We began packing. Good luck persisted, and that week we sold our house. After two years on the market without a nibble, this was incredible.

We bought a new home in Denton, and I was promoted to staff officer in charge of poultry-slaughter training materials. In this job I use my experience as an inspector and as an instructor to develop training materials such as lesson plans, booklets, modules, handouts, and even video and slide presentations for our inspectors. This information is used by instructors in our training center, field trainers, state inspectors, poultry industry personnel, and some veterinary colleges. Many people depend on me for accurate information.

Occasionally I serve on a task force to deal with a troublesome inspection problem. Some are routine, but others are very interesting, like our project involving osteomyelitis [a bone infection] in turkeys. I was on a team that developed a means to diagnose and prevent turkeys with osteomyelitis from reaching the consumer. As part of this team, I traveled across the United States to investigate the problem and worked closely with our Washington staff to write the government position paper that introduced stringent new inspection procedures. Although new procedures ensure safe food for the consumer, they create a headache for the poultry industry until it gallantly adjusts to our rules.

The government produced a video to help inspectors recognize osteomyelitis and handle infected carcasses. I wrote the script and was expert adviser to the camera crew and video editor. I thoroughly enjoyed this project because I used so many of my skills, from diagnostician to scriptwriter.

Once in a while I narrate a script for a training tape or video. My first time in a recording booth was intimidating. Eventually I learned how to make good recordings. Sometimes I think about cutting a demo tape and marketing myself as a medical narrator. Maybe someday I will.

My present job is a stimulating mixture of speaking, writing, a little theatrics, and a little teaching.

In the slaughter plants and now, politics has never kept me from doing what had to be done. Fortunately there is less politics in meat and poultry inspection than in other areas. I don't believe any politician wants to be accused of endangering the public's health or compromising its safe food supply. The agency I work for trains me to do a better job because it wants me to succeed.

Work is a game, albeit at times a serious one. All games have their rules. I learn them, then try to enjoy the action and keep things in the proper perspective. With government rules, the plays may take longer, but with patience a lot can get accomplished.

Women in government are paid the same as men for the same type of job. The federal system bends over backward to promote and train capable women. We are still underrepresented, but the gap is slowly narrowing. It pleases me that professional women managers in my agency perform as well as male managers by using their feminine style. They avoid being trapped into behaving like men. I and most of these women are probably what people refer to as women's libbers, but that doesn't mean we regard men as enemies. Every successful woman I know gets along well with both men and women, just as does every successful man. Being male or female isn't an issue.

A great fringe benefit of my job is twenty-six days a year paid vacation. My husband's work requires travel, sometimes to alluring places. If he is headed for Hawaii or Australia, I keep him company. If he goes to Newark, I stay home.

We also arrange pleasure trips to Europe, Mexico, and the Caribbean. Our biggest adventure, in May of 1987, was a three-week trip to mainland China. I was not eager to go, but Len talked me into it. His father had been a Swedish merchant marine, and Len grew up hearing stories about his dad's travels in China. I agreed to go only if we took a top-of-the-line tour that stayed at the best accommodations. On vacation, I like luxury.

Experienced travelers advised us to bring a supply of antibiotics, tissues, Handi-Wipes, plastic cutlery, and other "survival" items. Stepping off the plane in Canton was like stepping into a different world, and I will always remember the overwhelming sights, smells, and sounds of that fascinating land.

The other thing I'll always remember is to be grateful for being born in the United States, where life is so easy and comfortable. Although conditions in China's cities were vastly improved from just a few years ago, they lacked many things that we Americans consider bare necessities. No private citizen had a refrigerator; in fact, very few food stores had them. Although food was plentiful in the marketplace, I had to turn off my food-safety-and-hygiene mind to tour the open market. Poultry was sold live, or sometimes a dozen carcasses were laid on a dirty wood plank in the hot sun to wait for buyers. No animal part was wasted, and some parts were hard to identify. The Chinese people ate them all. Food varies considerably from one part of China to another, depending on the grains and animals raised. Rice is common in one location, wheat in another, and so forth.

Cleanliness was uncommon everywhere, which after a while was depressing. Everything was dingy or dirty. Attractive buildings were frequently covered with a layer of grime from severe air pollution. We used public rest rooms only as a last resort. Even government-operated planes looked as if they hadn't been cleaned for decades.

I was shocked by the realization that in a totalitarian state I had no rights as an individual. On one memorable plane trip our group got a taste of life under government control. We boarded the plane, thinking we would end up in a city in eastern China. Instead we landed in central China, thousands of miles from our destination. The government apparently altered the plane's route in midair.

The reason for the detour was never clear, but I will always remember the eight-hour layover in a small, dirty, isolated airport. No one knew when we would be allowed to leave. For four hours our tour guide tried to phone Beijing to arrange for another plane. We were told that in the big city there were only a small number of phones, perhaps twelve thousand, creating an endless busy signal.

We prayed for rescue, but we decided to eat because it might be twelve hours before our next meal. The restaurant across from the airport was supposedly the best in town. Our guide told the cooks to prepare a deluxe meal for important guests. From all the activity and attention, I'm sure they did. Unfortunately, many of the ingredients were a mystery. The dishes and chopsticks were unwashed, the shabby decor was depressing, and our appetites vanished. An M.D. in our group produced a bottle of Scotch that he had carried over half of China. This was the moment we needed a drink. I'm sure the Chinese cooks are still talking about the crazy Americans who brought their own plastic forks and spoons, wiped their plates with Handi-Wipes, and drank Scotch.

On our way home we stopped briefly in Japan. All of us were thrilled to be in such a clean country. The restaurant near the airport provided white linen tablecloths and napkins, even waiters in white gloves.

Many good things about China impressed me. The Chinese people were friendly and often spoke coherent English, which they learned on state-run television and radio. In contrast to their surroundings, they were clean and neat. I never felt threatened by anyone, and I enjoyed our limited conversations.

Very poor, the Chinese people live in a country with enormous problems, not the least of which is a population of one billion. They are taking serious steps to stop population growth and improve agriculture, education, housing, and living conditions. Anyone who has studied the history of China can see the many accomplishments that have been made in a short time. Every Chinese person we talked with was aware of the country's improvements. They believed that someday they could catch up with the West.

I was impressed by the love and care given to children. Because couples are limited to one child, that child is very precious. If love, care, and gentle discipline are as important in producing good human beings as the experts say, the generation growing up in China today should be some of the finest human beings in history.

In some poor countries like Mexico, young children live on the streets, abandoned by their families at an age when they should be enjoying a secure childhood. Instead they are unwanted excess. In China we suffered no such sights. It seems odd that a country condemned by many for suppressing religion and individual freedom treats children better than some nations that profess high values.

My work with the federal government has taught me, in a broad sense, to understand and admire how a democracy works and what it takes to make our political system grind out useful accomplishments. I understand American business through the food industry, and foreign economics now make more sense. Still, I feel very naive. Soon I'll have lived a half century. When I was young, I planned to be very wise at this age. Instead I'm constantly amazed at what I don't know. Perhaps it is the promise of more wisdom that makes life so interesting. My husband and I still expect to discover new places, new people, and new ideas. ■

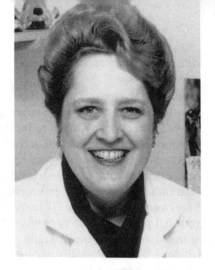

Barbara S. Stein

THE ROOM is crowded, every chair occupied, and latecomers lean against the walls or squat in corners. When lights signal a break in the lecture, people shift in their seats or stand to stretch, but few vacate the room, for fear of losing their place upon returning. As the lecturer, Barbara S. Stein, leaves the stage to set up visual aids for the next topic, twenty or so veterinarians crowd around her, bursting with questions.

An international authority on feline medicine and surgery, Stein has been a guest lecturer in South Africa, Japan, Switzerland, and Israel, as well as nearly every state in the United States. Other veterinarians seek her knowledge and advice. She speaks not from some ivory tower of the academic world but from expertise learned in medical and surgical practice at her own Chicago Cat Clinic. A prolific writer, she is known by pet owners for her *Book of the Cat* and is recognized by veterinarians for her chapters contributed to professional texts. She is a member of numerous advisory boards and committees as well as a consultant to industry and zoos.

In 1966 Stein earned her doctor of veterinary medicine degree from the College of Veterinary Medicine at Ohio State University in Columbus. She has been a member of the American Association of Feline Practitioners since its inception and has held every office, including that of president. Stein is also a member of the State of Illinois Veterinary Examining Board and serves on the advisory committee to the National Board of Veterinary Medical Examiners. In 1987 she became the first woman to serve on the veterinary advisory committee of the Food and Drug Administration. She is one of ten clinicians elected to the Council on Veterinary Services of the American Veterinary Medical Association, serving her term until 1994. Stein received the 1986 American Animal Hospital Association Carnation Award for Outstanding Achievement in Feline Medicine and Surgery and the 1987 Distinguished Alumnus Award from the Ohio State University College of Veterinary Medicine.

Such recognition has not come easily. Stein's life story reflects a determination to pursue her goals despite rebuffs and setbacks. Her initial application to veterinary school was rejected. The bank refused her a loan for her clinic because "a single woman was a poor financial risk." She was warned that cats alone couldn't support a private practice. Yet driven by her love for animals, especially cats, Stein adhered to the course she set for herself at age eight, when she decided to spend her life healing "broken animals."

■

A belief once prevailed that real men don't own cats. Many people still regard cats as second-class pet citizens. When I first entered practice, veterinarians with this attitude told me, "Be careful what you do with a sick cat. After all, it's only a cat, and the owners might not want to spend the money on it." I didn't understand why a ten-pound Persian might be valued less than a ten-pound poodle.

Despite this advice, in 1975 I risked opening my Chicago Cat Clinic. At that time, very few veterinarians limited their practice to cats. I was risking not only my resources but those of my parents. My father and mother offered their house as collateral for a loan that enabled me to rent and renovate a building.

The old attitudes are vanishing today, and cats have become pets favored by both sexes. They're popular because they're well-suited to the yuppie life-style. It is difficult for dual-career families to provide the space, exercise, and care required by a dog. A cat doesn't pollute the environment and doesn't tie an owner down in the same way as a dog.

I grew up with my older brother, Robert, in northwest Chicago. Because my father owned a small hardware business, he understood the importance of self-reliance. When the time came for me to start my own business, he encouraged me. His guidance was the single most important factor enabling me to gain any degree of success. He planted within me both business and people sense.

My parents, who respected all living things, allowed us to keep various birds, turtles, lizards, rabbits, tropical fish, dogs, and cats. My mother drew the line with rodents. That's probably why my first pet when I was away at college was a hamster.

On visits to my uncle's farm near Verona, Wisconsin, I encountered larger animals. Once, unknown to my uncle, my cousin Art sneaked me into the farrowing house to witness the birth of baby pigs. My uncle disapproved of a young girl being exposed to the realities of farm-animal reproduction. However, after I graduated from veterinary school, my uncle lost his reservations about such exposure. When I visited as a real veterinarian (and for free), he asked me to palpate a cow for pregnancy using an old obstetrical glove left years ago by a veterinarian.

I decided to become a veterinarian at age eight. Encouraged by my parents, I assumed that everyone would be supportive. It came as a complete surprise that others would try to discourage me. My high school adviser dismissed such aspirations as foolishness. She explained, "Nice Jewish girls do not become veterinarians."

During my senior year I attended preveterinary day at the University of Illinois College of Veterinary Medicine in Urbana. A faculty member asked, "Well, why do you want to be a veterinarian? And don't tell me it's because you love animals." It puzzled me then that love for animals was an inappropriate answer, and it still upsets me when members of the profession are reluctant to accept that response from aspiring candidates. If more students became veterinarians because of their love for animals, our profession would be even better.

This love for animals made me question, however, if I could perform euthanasia, a task required of a veterinarian. On a day I remember vividly, I had to have my beloved boxer put to sleep. As I held her, she quickly and painlessly slipped into death. I understood then that euthanasia was a kind and gentle solution to an animal's suffering. When an animal cannot be helped, a veterinarian has not only the right but also the responsibility to perform euthanasia. It is the last act of love for which an owner should be responsible.

Although neither my mother nor my father had graduated from high school, they had given my brother and me the incentive to pursue professional degrees. Robert chose engineering mechanics, and my goal at the time of high school graduation was clear. I chose Ohio State University for preprofessional study partly because it had graduated more women veterinarians than any other school in the nation.

Upon completing my two years, I applied for admission into the College of Veterinary Medicine. Before my appointment with the selection committee, fellow students warned me to avoid wearing anything feminine, such as nail polish or jewelry. They felt that token women who were accepted had to be "one of the boys." The best candidates, I felt, would be students academically qualified, whether female or male. However, I didn't intend to take any chances. I wore a plain brown plaid suit to the interview and tried to minimize my femininity. Regardless of my drab appearance and my competitive grade point average, my application was rejected.

It never occurred to me to give up. A year later, I again applied to Ohio State. With another year of course work and a high grade point average, I felt sure of acceptance. I wore an ultraconservative blue suit to the interview. The rejection notice came just as I finished packing to return home to Chicago. I couldn't believe I'd been rejected again.

I immediately phoned for an appointment with the veterinary school dean. Glancing at my low-cut peasant dress, I thought, I can't wear this. But everything was packed and at the moment, I felt that what I wore was unimportant.

That visit with the dean discouraged me from thinking I'd ever be accepted into veterinary school. I turned to Dr. William Tyznik, my animal-science professor and adviser. A College of Agriculture staff member, he also taught nutrition at the College of Veterinary Medicine. Each year he recommended one student to the Veterinary College Selection Board. Almost all of the students he recommended were women. Most of them later successfully practiced veterinary medicine.

Dr. Tyznik would try to help, but I had little hope. At home my application to medical school was quickly accepted. However, with my heart set on veterinary school, I was depressed about the thought of starting the fall term in medicine. A subsequent notice of acceptance as an Ohio State veterinary school alternate gave little encouragement. I felt that my chances for replacing one of four or five women who might drop out were slim.

On August 2, 1962, I received notification of my acceptance into the College of Veterinary Medicine at Ohio State University. I started my course work on September 24, my birthday, as one of four women in a class of seventy-two freshmen.

I gratefully took up veterinary student life. Neither the faculty nor the students exhibited discrimination against women. I felt an unexpected camaraderie among classmates, both male and female.

My goal remained unchanged—to "fix animals." As graduation approached, I interviewed at small-animal hospitals. In 1966, with the Vietnam War escalating and eligible men being drafted, I was offered a job at Berwyn Animal Hospital, a small-animal practice in a western suburb of Chicago. I joined a staff of three male veterinarians.

Because I liked cats and cat owners, I began to see most of the cat cases. I felt that if the client cared enough to bring the cat to the hospital, he or she cared enough to pay for treatment. Dr. Herb Lederer, my employer, allowed me every Thursday afternoon to pursue my interest in feline medicine and surgery, with the stipulation that at the end of the year I give lectures on feline medicine to Chicago veterinarians.

At this time, feline practitioners were almost unheard-of. Most research and textbooks were devoted to canine medicine and surgery. I read textbooks and journals, visited practitioners with special interest or expertise in feline medicine, and enrolled in courses concerning cats.

Close monitoring of my patients contributed to my knowledge. With owner permission, I performed a necropsy on every cat that died and submitted tissues for histopathological examination. Under the microscope, tissues often revealed more disease than expected. I kept extensive records of cases and made photographs and slides of interesting cases for use in my lectures.

At my first lecture before colleagues, I was apprehensive. But people came back for repeat seminars. Veterinarians started referring their difficult cat cases to me. I was asked to lecture at veterinary association meetings. After a while, I received a financial honorarium for these efforts.

In 1969 Berwyn Animal Hospital moved into a new building with considerably more space to accommodate the staff of six veterinarians and five visiting specialists. By now we were the largest veterinary practice in Chicago.

After seven years, I decided to pursue my dream of living and practicing in California. With this goal in mind, I had passed the California boards soon after graduation. With prospects of my purchasing a practice in southern California, my parents put their house up for sale in anticipation of moving with me to the West Coast.

I made seven trips to California during the next five months to negotiate the purchase of a practice. Finally, the time for finalizing the sale arrived. With my belongings loaded on a trailer, I flew out with my father, my accountant, and my attorney. We sat in a large room with the owner of the practice and his attorney. After signing the documents, I passed them to the veterinarian. He picked up a pen and hesitated. Finally he said, "I think I want to search my soul before I sign these papers."

Disappointed and broke, I returned home to search my own

soul. Out of desperation and economic necessity, I started a house-call service from my home. Without advertising, the practice quickly grew. Surgeries were performed in the clinic of a friend and colleague, Dr. Robert McLain. Soon 80 percent of my patients were cats. In addition to clients with felines, I catered to handicapped pet owners such as the blind with seeing-eye dogs, to elderly clients, to women with small children, and to dual-career families.

After working out of my car for two years, I located a building near a pleasant residential area in northwest Chicago. With plans and projections for an animal hospital in hand, I began to look for a bank loan. Seven banks later, I was no closer to securing financing than when I began my search. Bankers were reluctant to lend money for a practice devoted solely to cats. They seemed put off by a single woman wanting a loan. Frustrated, I asked a loan officer if I would have better luck securing a loan if I were married to a house husband. His smug response was, "Marriage to anyone is better than being single if you want a loan." It is hard to argue with that kind of thinking. Eventually, with a loan from my parents, I rented the building I had selected, and we began renovations.

My father, as general contractor for repairs, was working late one night at the clinic with an electrician. I was painting walls in the next room when I heard him ask my dad, "Don't you think you are taking a hell of a risk on your daughter?" My father replied, "I've taken risks all of my life. What safer risk can be taken than one for my own daughter?" I've always cherished his response.

Working together, my father and I were proud of the results of our remodeling. We knew every square inch of the building. Today my employees are amazed that I can tell them the location of individual studs and screws.

Much time, work, and research went into the clinic design. At least 25 percent of the total building cost went into an elaborate ventilation system that allows fifteen air exchanges per hour in each animal ward. This avoids recirculation of air and eliminates odors and the spread of feline respiratory diseases. If I had designed a traditional dog-cat hospital, the expense would have been far less than for my cat clinic. I am still irritated by people who believe that cat practice is a low-cost investment.

During that first lean year, my father would walk into the hospital with a check for five hundred or a thousand dollars. "Take it," he would say. "You can't practice scared." Eventually, my parents were paid back in full for their loans. A plaque inside the front door of the clinic reads:

Chicago Cat Clinic
Dedicated to My Parents
Julius and Martha Stein
March 1975

Although my father died in 1984, he lived long enough to enjoy some of my successes. He was proud when I was asked to lecture all over the United States and overseas.

With the financial success of Chicago Cat Clinic, I bought the building, assuring us long-term security of location. I like to think that although I am an integral part of the clinic, if I died tomorrow, the clinic would survive.

Our staff of nineteen employees includes three other associate veterinarians, five veterinary technicians, an office manager, receptionists, bookkeepers, and animal caretakers. At present the staff is female except for one veterinary technician.

I don't think it matters whether the staff is male or female. What matters is that an individual acts and dresses professionally and communicates well with both staff members and clients.

Because of the large staff, we can accommodate each other for vacations and continuing education programs. All of our veterinarians attend at least one major professional meeting each year, and we share our learning. The longer we're out of school, the faster we must pedal to stay abreast of the overwhelming amount of new knowledge.

The American Association of Feline Practitioners is a professional organization created by veterinarians with a special interest in feline medicine. A member from the start, I have held every association office. Our goals are to advance continuing education in feline medicine and practice and to raise the standard of feline practice so that eventually we will have board certification status.

This year the association sponsored with Cornell University an intensive week-long seminar offering the forefront of knowledge in feline medicine and surgery. Worldwide interest in feline medicine is increasing, as attested by the 150 or more people attending the seminar from the United States and several foreign countries.

Sponsored by Kyoritsu Shoji Company, a Japanese veterinary business, I was the first guest speaker to present a program in Japan strictly about cats. It was an honor to be asked to speak in a conservative, male-dominated country. Among the one thousand veterinarians in the Tokyo audience, 5 percent were women. The only Japanese women who own practices are those married to practicing veterinarians. In speaking with several women, I found their concerns to be similar to those of women veterinarians in this country—finding the time and energy necessary to balance home, family, and career obligations.

I had not dreamed that my profession would offer such wonderful opportunities for travel. I have presented a program about feline medicine in Israel and lectured to the South Africa Veterinary Clinicians Group. Overseas speaking engagements are all-expense trips with stopovers in cities like London, Rio de Janeiro, and Lucerne. Although the lecture circuit takes me from the practice, my clients remain loyal. They are interested in my travels and tolerate my absences with good grace.

The popularity of *The Book of Cats* has been fun. I am amused by pet owners who ask for my autograph and then proceed to quote from the book. If I'm not careful in what I say, they accuse me of contradicting my published words.

The devotion of dedicated owners to their pets and the will of certain animals to survive always amaze me. Take Tar Baby, for example. Late one night I received a call from a woman who had just witnessed a group of boys pouring tar on a cat and burying it alive. What should she do? she asked. I told her, "Go unbury the cat, and bring it in immediately."

The lady arrived at the hospital carrying a pathetic black glob from which stared two glazed eyes. We treated the cat for shock and later softened the tar with many applications of mineral oil until we were able to remove much of it by clipping or washing with warm, soapy water.

I didn't think the creature would survive the night. However, showing a will to live, Tar Baby slowly improved during her three-week stay in the hospital. Her lady rescuer continued to nurse her at home for many more months. Today the only evidence of Tar Baby's life-threatening experience is her name.

Recently, I examined a tiny kitten born with both inguinal and umbilical hernias. When the kitten was six weeks old, I worked for two hours in surgery to reconstruct his abdominal wall. A month later, the owner brought the kitten in for vaccinations. He was a perfectly normal, ornery little fellow. When I showed him to the staff, no one recognized the kitten until I asked them to feel his belly. The internal stainless steel sutures were easily felt. Those who had worked so hard with that kitten oohed and aahed when they realized it was the baby with the hernia.

Such a moment brings tears to my eyes, not just for the kitten but for the joy and satisfaction experienced by the staff. That's what veterinary medicine is all about—fixing broken animals. The day that we don't get a little adrenalin surge after a sick or injured animal is healed is the day we really do have burnout and need to reevaluate our priorities.

One of my priorities in practice is to continue to learn new and better ways of treating my patients. Sometimes I work with university or industrial veterinarians to monitor feline diseases or to aid the evolution of veterinary medical products.

Companies that market pet food, pharmaceuticals, or equipment for the pet health industry often ask my advice about the development of new products. In a recent study funded by a major veterinary company in conjunction with the University of California at Davis, we were to determine the frequency of taurine deficiency in the average household cat. A low level or complete absence in a cat's diet of the amino acid taurine can lead to degeneration of the retina of the eye, cardiomyopathy, and reproductive failure.

With the owner's consent, we drew blood for analysis and performed a retinal eye exam on every tenth cat entering the hospital. Through these findings and information collected on the cat's dietary history, we hope to gain valuable information helpful to the pet food industry.

I have worked to develop a liquid diet for critically ill or injured animals, and I have evaluated laboratory tests for thyroid function and for feline immunodeficiency virus. These experiences are exciting because I can collaborate with company representatives and with other veterinarians to find what will or won't work and what the needs are of veterinarians and potential product consumers.

I am probably away from my practice 30 percent of the time. At least half of that time is spent serving on editorial boards for veterinary publications, on professional committees, and on advisory councils. I serve on these boards and committees because I am proud to be a veterinarian and excited about what is going on in the profession. I also believe that we each have a responsibility to give back more than we received from our profession, our college, and those who believed in us.

Woody Hayes, the well-known Ohio State football coach, had a favorite saying: "You can never pay back, but you can pay ahead." Although I can't repay those who helped me, I can help others with my involvement and interest in veterinary medicine. This is an exciting time to be a veterinarian because our profession is facing so many changes and issues. As a member of the advisory committee for the Food and Drug Administration, I hear major concerns about drug residues in milk and the carcasses of food animals. The FDA has traced cases of sulfa and antibiotic residues in animals that have been treated improperly. The abuse rarely involves a veterinarian. In most cases, a layperson gives the animal an injection of penicillin purchased at a feedstore and then sells the milk or carcass without observing the antibiotic withdrawal time.

The number of unwanted pets euthanized each year in this country is a major concern of veterinarians and others who care about animals. At a national conference on the ecology of the problem of surplus dogs and cats, a presenter gave some staggering statistics. If every veterinarian alive today devoted five days a week to performing surgery to neuter dogs and cats, the population of unwanted animals would be reduced by only 10 percent. Surgery is not the answer. Chemical contraception for animals would be helpful, but the prime need in this country is the education of the pet-owning public.

I am one of ten elected clinicians who make up the Veterinary Services Council of the American Veterinary Medical Association (AVMA). We evaluate professional issues facing veterinary practitioners and make recommendations to the AVMA executive board about policies.

For example, a veterinarian wrote for advice about a new hospital he was building. Hospital zoning had already been approved, but his city passed new zoning restrictions for handicapped employees that would require major expensive renovations to construction already in progress. The council wrote a letter supporting the veterinarian's original plans. We felt that access for handicapped clients was a legitimate requirement, but that renovation of the entire hospital to accommodate a potential handicapped employee was too stringent a restriction. Problems such as this start with the individual veterinarian but have an impact on all of us.

Government restrictions make it more difficult to practice veterinary medicine legally, ethically, and morally. I have a lawyer, an accountant, and an office manager. It takes all three to keep the business adhering to government regulations. Practicing veterinarians become frustrated when they can no longer practice quality veterinary medicine. They are consumed by paperwork involved in operating a business.

Regulations that govern the licensing of practicing veterinarians are now being scrutinized by most states. As a member of the State of Illinois Veterinary Examining Board and the advisory committee to the National Board of Veterinary Medical Examiners, I foresee changes in licensing requirements. As veterinary schools test the waters with specialty training, boards will be forced to consider changes.

Limited licensing makes sense. Most people who have been out of school any length of time have great difficulty passing a broad exam that covers every facet of veterinary medicine. These people are also the least likely to stray from their area of expertise.

Since I graduated, the number of women entering veterinary medicine has dramatically increased. This is a wonderful career for women because it allows us to capitalize on natural traits of empathy and nurturance. However, I am concerned about the lack of business interest in many of today's young women. I encourage veterinary students to take business courses and seek advice from financial organizations supporting women in business. I also encourage young women to dress and act in a professional manner. Dress alone doesn't make or break anyone, but it is part of a successful image. Both sexes, as veterinarians, should have confidence in what they are offering and charge what their work is worth.

Young graduates who want it all—career, marriage, children—should go out and try for it. They may have to reroute along the way, but that shouldn't prevent them from pursuing their goals. I know two women veterinarians with young children who jointly own a small-animal practice. They recently chose to hire a full-time male veterinarian, so they both might work only half-time.

There are times when I wish that I had children and a good marriage as well as my career. However, family obligations might preclude opportunities to travel and lecture. Involvement in professional activities is a luxury I enjoy because I have none of these personal commitments.

My goal is to continue learning. I'd like to return to school and study for a law degree. I'd like to learn foreign languages. I want to continue my travels and spend more time with my hobbies of gardening, music, and photography.

However, I don't foresee leaving veterinary practice. I

might decrease my hours by half, but I will continue helping animals. I believe the old adage that says you must have an essential belief in yourself and enjoy what you do. I enjoy veterinary medicine immensely. It is a wonderful profession.   ■

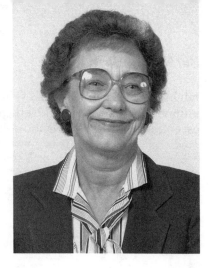

Virginia M. Streets

IN THE sleepy, picturesque Dutch community of Lynden, Washington, Virginia M. Streets carved out her niche as veterinarian, wife, mother, musician, and community and church volunteer. For forty years she and the people of Lynden have shared the type of unity best demonstrated in rural small-town America.

Streets maintains balance in life by combining her profession, talents, and family. The same quiet, hospitable woman who skillfully ministers to her neighbors' pets also sings tenor and plays the piano and organ at the Lynden United Methodist Church; composed an ode titled "Dr. Pill and Dr. Pull" to the local physician and dentist upon their retirement; serves as Democratic precinct committeewoman; and represented her county's six chapters of PEO (women's philanthropic education organization) at the organization's international convention in Orlando in 1987. In her roles of mother and grandmother, Streets has provided the music for Bluebird programs, served as perennial room mother, and assisted as booster for Cub Scouts and for Little League baseball and basketball.

At first glance, Streets, a seasoned

veterinarian with more than forty-five years of practice experience, seems reserved. However, closer observation reveals an individual who approaches life with humor, grit, and bulldog tenacity. When her seventh-grade classmates reacted with ridicule toward her aspiration to become a veterinarian, Streets became more determined. When a veterinary school professor demanded that Streets, the only woman in the class, chew tobacco with the men, she did that too. When the farmers of Lynden, many fresh from the old country, asked if she had learned her animal-doctoring trade from her husband, Dr. Ernie Streets, she replied, "No, I taught him."

But none of her tough roles defined the type of woman Streets was or is. She won the envy of her junior high and high school classmates with her talents in music and by dating the popular captain of the football team. During the rigors of veterinary school classes in an old building called the Vet Shack, she maintained her skill in the social graces by playing with the Washington State University Symphony Orchestra and living in the Alpha Gamma Delta sorority house. And throughout her husband's long, progressive illness and then death, she maintained a hopeful and optimistic outlook toward life. Streets credits her strength during the years of Ernie's declining health to the love and care of the people of Lynden, the comfort she receives from music, and the challenges of her profession.

Streets was named Outstanding Woman Veterinarian of the Year in 1985 by the Association for Women Veterinarians. Still practicing small-animal medicine part-time, she says, "To me, veterinary practice is just as exciting today as it was forty years ago. I have such wonderful memories and no regrets."

■

My life here in Lynden has been intertwined with family, profession, and community. Ernie and I moved to this small farming town in 1950 and set up Streets Veterinary Hospital in a building that also served as our home. The practice was small, and we did everything ourselves. I saw small animals and took telephone calls for Ernie while he was on the road seeing large-animal patients. Our two daughters cleaned the kennels and exercised the dogs.

One of the advantages of a family business is that I was home when the girls got out of school. I could balance a baby on one hip and give a rabies shot to a farmer's dog or do the monthly statements while playing "office" with the children.

Lynden is such a small community that everyone knew where to find us, and because we lived at the hospital, they came and rang the doorbell at all hours of the day or night. In the early days we had a local telephone operator who could always track us down if, for example, I was at school for a PTA meeting or Ernie was having coffee at the local cafe or getting a haircut. If we went out for an evening or a weekend, we called Thelma, the telephone operator, and told her where we were going. Today the veterinarians I work with hire an answering service and carry beepers. Things have really changed in the forty-five years I've been a veterinarian.

Veterinary medicine was not a profession that young girls considered when I was growing up. We were pretty much restricted to three jobs—nursing, teaching, and secretarial work. In 1935 when I was in the seventh grade, I was required to take and pass the state examination. The test covered everything we had learned in the seven years of grammar school. One of my teachers who was coaching us for the exam told us that the test also asked if we had decided our life's work. My teacher encouraged us to think about our future so we could respond intelligently.

I went home and discussed my future with my parents and younger brother. My father was an architect, and my mother, who had met and married my father during World War I, had worked as a secretary to help support my uncle through architecture school at the University of Washington. Later, my brother followed in the family footsteps by pursuing architecture as a career, so I was totally immersed in the design and building trade. I would probably have chosen that career field, just because of its familiarity and my reluctance to choose one of the traditional women's jobs, but my parents said, "You like to work with animals, so why don't you become a veterinarian?"

We owned all kinds of animals, including horses, goats, chickens, rabbits, dogs, and cats and lived on a small acreage on Mercer Island. The island is located in lower Puget Sound and in those days was just a wilderness, a refuge of wild and domestic animals. If a small bird or squirrel or one of our animals was injured, I was always the one to take care of it. When my parents suggested that I become an animal doctor, I thought it was a good idea.

When the state examination rolled around, I designated that my life's work would be in veterinary medicine. Everyone laughed at me, and I felt humiliated. I was very sensitive and bashful at that age, but the more they teased and laughed, the more determined I became.

During high school, I lost some of my shyness. I felt like the ugly duckling who became a swan when I finally got those awful braces off my teeth and had my straight hair permed. My esteem went up another notch when I began dating the football captain. However, I never lost my dream of becoming a veterinarian. Later, there were many times, especially during my first year in veterinary school, when I thought I had made a big mistake.

I started preveterinary studies in 1940 at Washington State University in Pullman. I joined a sorority my second year there and lived in the sorority house three of the four years that I spent at WSU. Alpha Gamma Delta deserves a lot of credit for accepting me. I know there were a few times when they wondered why they had taken a veterinary student.

Often I'd have to participate in a sorority skit immediately after class. I'd ask my veterinary classmates for creative ideas. The year we were in anatomy lab, one of my classmates suggested taking a cow's eye and displaying it for the sorority group. I put the big brown eye, intact with all its muscles sticking out like spikes, on a china plate. My opening speech went something like, "Here's looking at you, folks."

Another time, I demonstrated vital organs using a shiny pink fetal pig. My sorority sisters received a real education in anatomy. My saving graces were that I could play the piano and was comfortable with social etiquette. I still have friends from the sorority, and when we met for our forty-fifth reunion in Newport Beach, California, one of my sisters mentioned the eye skit.

I obtained my B.S. degree in January 1944 and my D.V.M. in September 1944, four years after I started college at WSU. Those were the war years, and we went to school year-round to keep the fellows from being drafted. My veterinary school class started with thirty-seven men and three women students. Thirty-five of us were graduated, and I was the only woman to finish. I was about the ninth woman to graduate as a veterinarian from WSU. The first woman finished in 1933, I think. I was told that the teachers liked to have one or two women in each class to settle things down. Well, if we settled them down, it was undetectable.

The building that housed the veterinary school, called the Vet Shack, was ancient and terrible. Sanitation was not a priority. Everything, including surgery, was pretty primitive then, and everyone, professors and students alike, seemed to act accordingly. I remember being told that in order to graduate from anatomy class, I had to chew tobacco. I said, "I can do that." And I did. I wasn't about to let the guys or the professor get away with intimidating me.

We moved to a new building at the start of my sophomore year. The new surroundings were clean and airy, and the attitude of everyone changed for the better. The old anatomy professor who had insisted that I chew tobacco resigned. The new atmosphere just wasn't his thing anymore.

When I first started veterinary school, I was told at least once a week that I was taking the place of a man. Several of my professors said, "You may graduate and that's questionable, but you'll just get married. At most, you will practice six months." I was determined that I was going to graduate and that I was going to practice in order to prove all those critics wrong.

After a while, my classmates accepted me and became very

protective of me. Because I was small and petite, they always insisted in large-animal clinics that I work on the goats and ponies rather than the cattle and draft horses. I was excused if a stallion was brought in for breeding because they were embarrassed to have me in the barn during that activity.

While I was in veterinary school, I fell in love with a student majoring in business who lived at the Beta house. He told me that because I was going to be a veterinarian, our relationship could never lead to marriage. I was heartbroken and decided then that I was going to have to marry a veterinarian. No one else would understand.

Finding a marriage partner was not what I had in mind when I started work at Seattle Veterinary Hospital soon after graduation from veterinary school. Yet that's where I met Ernie, my future husband.

Dr. E. A. Ehmer, who had quite a reputation for being a progressive small-animal practitioner, owned Seattle Veterinary Hospital. He already employed one veterinarian and wasn't looking for another, especially a woman. However, I was most insistent and told him that I would work for practically nothing. That appealed to his conservative nature, and I was hired.

I learned more about small-animal medicine in the year with Dr. Ehmer than I learned in veterinary school. He did all of the spays and neuters for the local humane society, and I don't think he ever charged for one of them. That was one area where I was allowed to hone my surgical skills. The injectable anesthetic sodium pentobarbital had just come out, and he teased me about wanting to use it. He would say, "Oh, you new graduates. You always want to use those injectable things that you can't get back once they are injected. I never lose an animal because I use ether."

Dr. Ehmer was a real pioneer and far ahead of his time. He performed diaphragmatic hernia surgery long before the days of gas anesthesia. A person, usually me, had to operate a hand bellows attached to an endotracheal tube to keep the patient breathing while the chest was open. He also developed the Ehmer sling, which is a bandage technique used for luxations of the hip and formerly used for fractures of the femur and humerus. However, the work for which he is most recognized is the Kirschner bone-pinning system which he developed with Don Kirschner and Dr. Fred Cummings.

Don and Bill Kirschner owned a manufacturing plant west of Seattle and developed the bone pins there. They were mainly interested in the human application of the pins but enticed Dr.

Ehmer to test the pinning system in dogs first. The idea at that time was to reduce the fracture and maintain bone apposition through the use of half pins above and below the fracture site that were connected with an extension bar.

I had been at Seattle Veterinary Hospital only a short period of time when this fellow who had been wounded in the war showed up to work through the summer. That fellow who soon became my fellow was Ernie Streets, and he left Seattle to begin preveterinary studies at WSU in the fall. After Ernie left for college, my work didn't seem nearly as interesting.

I made plans to visit Ernie in Pullman and attend a WSU football game. Before the game, I made a brief visit to the veterinary school and, much to my surprise, was offered a job as instructor in the small-animal clinic. Ernie and I talked it over and decided that I should accept the position and stay in Pullman. We eloped instead of going to the football game.

I started as the assistant to the man in charge of small-animal clinics. That individual left the next semester, and I was suddenly in charge of the entire small-animal section, including surgery. We had a moderate caseload, but all of my students had the opportunity to perform six or seven spays before graduation. I also utilized my experiences at Dr. Ehmer's hospital and encouraged orthopedic surgery, including intramedullary pinning, which was a new technique at that time.

My students, who eventually included Ernie's class, were a close-knit group. Most were veterans and shared similar experiences. They often came to our house to study or just to talk. Even though Ernie died in 1973, I am still invited to his class reunions and am still considered part of that family of friends and colleagues.

I have a lot of memories about my teaching days. At one point, I decided that I should be teaching grooming techniques. There were no formal schools for dog grooming, and I thought this might be an additional source of income for my students. I remember this one student, his eyes filled with horror, who ran over to tell me that his dog's ear fell off when he started clipping it. It was a cocker spaniel with a rubber band around the base of its ear; the only thing holding the ear to the dog was its fur. I had an awful time trying to get that student to pick up the clippers after that episode.

Our older daughter was born while Ernie and I were in Pullman, and I stayed at home during Ernie's junior year in veterinary school. However, the summer before his senior year, we decided to work during the break for a classmate of mine who needed help testing cattle during a brucellosis outbreak.

Bleeding cattle was a new experience for both Ernie and me. We started out at 4 A.M. to pick up the baby-sitter, and once we had the baby settled, we drove to the farm where we'd be working for the day. We had decided on a division of labor; Ernie would draw the blood, and I would do the paperwork.

I remember one of our first jobs, which was to bleed a herd of eighty cows. This was in the days of old-time manger-style barns, so Ernie and the farmer crawled into the manger, caught the first cow to be bled, and the farmer held the cow with nose tongs while Ernie attempted to hit its vein. Well, Ernie was new at this, and things were progressing pretty slowly. After negotiating about forty mangers and coaxing out as many vials of the elusive blood, we noticed the farmer just sort of fading away. He mumbled something about his insulin shot before he passed out. We stopped and ministered to the farmer before proceeding with our work on the herd. That was the hard way to find out just how long it takes to bleed eighty cows under those conditions.

While we were working for my classmate, the veterinary school administration wired me an offer of more money to come back and teach another year. Before that, I think they thought they could get away with paying me less because I had to be there while Ernie was in school. I accepted the job but was hesitant about going back because I would have to teach my husband's class.

Teaching a class with one's spouse in it shouldn't happen to a dog. Ernie and I had worked together at Dr. Ehmer's, and he had helped me develop the surgery class syllabus. He already knew where I was coming from on everything I had to teach. He deserved a good grade, but I was worried that if I gave him an A, the other students would feel that he had an unfair advantage. If I gave him less than an A, he would be mad because he obviously knew the material. It was an awful dilemma, and I finally solved it by giving him an A-minus.

After Ernie graduated in 1950, we moved to Lynden and established our combination hospital and home. In time, we added normal living quarters and enlarged the hospital area. We spent twenty-one years at that location. When we first opened the hospital, farmers often asked me if I had learned my trade from my husband. I'd say, "No, I taught him."

Our clients just couldn't seem to get the idea that we were both doctors, so Ernie became Dr. Streets and I became Mrs.

Streets. I still run into some of that thinking today, and I always make a point at the hospital to refer to myself as Dr. Streets.

The farmers were hesitant about discussing large-animal reproductive problems with me. However, women were most often the ones who brought in the small animals, and they were comfortable with me. I've always thought it was a great advantage being a woman, because pets respond so well to women and are often intimidated by the gruffness of men.

Ernie and I worked long hours. He did all the large-animal work, and his territory was immense. When I wasn't busy with my own small-animal patients, I was on the telephone, calling him about his patients. During the twenty-one years that we owned the clinic, we hired only two employees, one who cleaned once a week and another who took care of the girls, did housework, cleaned kennels, and was like a right hand to me. The girls grew up to love animals, but they didn't want to have anything to do with veterinary medicine because of the long hours.

Lynden is a conservative community, but we had lots of exciting experiences during the sixties when hippies traveled through on their way to Canada. The town is only five miles from the border. I remember one night when the doorbell rang at 3 A.M. I got up to answer the door and was shocked to see this tall, bearded man with long hair and dressed in flowing white robes. I was half asleep and thought that I was finally meeting Jesus. However, this wasn't a religious experience. It was just a flower child, stopping by in the middle of the night for a five-dollar rabies vaccination for his dog. All dogs crossing the border had to be vaccinated against rabies.

At other times, people stopped in beat-up vans covered with graffiti and left with us birds and monkeys, which weren't allowed across the border. Sometimes they came back for them, and sometimes they didn't.

I could always be counted on to provide an exotic animal such as one of those monkeys for show-and-tell at the grade school. Our lives, professional and personal, mingled with the others who lived in this small community. The positive side was being surrounded by people who cared about us, but the down side was being tied down to the point of rarely escaping our professional obligations.

Ernie and I never got away together for vacations. When one of us was gone, the other worked to keep the practice going. Each summer, the children and I would cruise the San Juan Islands with my parents on their boat. Ernie and his friends would take an old bus they had converted into a motor home and go to eastern Washington for fall hunting season.

When Ernie became ill, our priorities totally changed, and we took some very nice trips together. We just locked the doors of the clinic and referred cases to other veterinarians. We would sometimes be gone a month or more at a time traveling in our small motor home. It was one of those now-or-never situations.

Ernie was hunting in eastern Washington when he had his first attack of what was later diagnosed as spinal cerebellar ataxia. That was in 1963, on the day President Kennedy was shot. Ernie was forty-three years old then. In 1973 he died, totally disabled.

Spinal cerebellar ataxia is an inherited degenerative disease that does not usually show up until the affected individual is forty to fifty years old. We already had our family by the time Ernie's illness became evident. Each child has a 50 percent chance of developing the disorder. Our older daughter is now in her early forties, and the disease is a constant worry for our family. I am sure that it has influenced my younger daughter to remain childless. My older daughter has two sons.

Ernie was able to practice with difficulty until 1971, when we sold the practice. The disease affected his balance, and he worked until he could no longer stand up. The farmers would have him come out to treat an animal and have to hold him up so he could work. Ernie, who had been a big, strong man, had spent his entire life outdoors, and it was so very hard for him to accept that he would eventually be confined to a wheelchair.

We finally hired Dr. Vern Pedersen and sold the practice to him a short time later. I continued to work for the new owner. Ernie wanted me to quit work and stay home with him. I just couldn't do that because my work helped to save my sanity during those extremely stressful years. I have always been a one-track person. At work I forget about everything else, and I was able to forget about Ernie's problems for a few hours each day. To compensate for my absence, I hired a good-looking woman to come in to visit with him while I was gone. Ernie didn't mind that at all!

I had such good neighbors and friends and the church and my music. All of these things helped me cope during those years. Our younger daughter lived at home, and although the situation was frustrating to all of us, we supported each other. Now people my age are all going through some type of loss. I've had mine, and I can go on to other things.

Streets Veterinary Hospital eventually became Kulshan Veterinary Hospital, and I have worked part-time for the new owners since 1971. The hospital has developed into a large practice with nine doctors. A new modern facility was built in 1975.

We certainly aren't a fire-engine practice anymore. The livestock industry is much more sophisticated, and veterinarians are called upon to offer additional services such as herd health work, nutritional counseling, and embryo transfer. The small-animal practice has also grown because the area is expanding. People are moving in from California and other areas to retire here.

I still enjoy practice. I love the contact with the clients, and I find the work stimulating. I like to instruct people about the care of their pets. If a new puppy or kitten comes in, I spend a lot of time talking with the owners about training, behavior problems, nutrition, and vaccination programs. Good communication builds loyalty and trust between veterinarian and client.

One of the reasons practice is never boring is that you can't predict what might be requested of you. I remember a man, a physician in fact, who came rushing into the office from Canada. He was carrying his dog in his arms and laid it gently down on the examination table and said, "Please help me. There is something wrong with this dog." Well, there certainly was something wrong. The dog was stone-dead and had been that way for hours. I think the man was disgusted with me because I couldn't bring his dog back to life.

Another time, a man came in with an old Labrador retriever that had been diagnosed as having cancer. The dog was in such bad shape that he couldn't hold his head up and just sort of melted onto the exam table. The owner told me that his dog had been such a wonderful pet that he just had to get a pup from him. I appeased the man, who was terribly agitated, by taking the old dog into the treatment room. I tried to get a semen sample by enticing the elderly canine with a bitch in heat, but the poor old fellow just looked up at me as if to say, "Are you crazy?" We never did get a pup out of that one.

Clients say the most interesting things. For example, one client told me, "This dog was just fine until a couple of days ago, and it suddenly became emancipated." Another told me, "This dog eats anything and everything. She's so gullible." It's real important to slow down enough to appreciate and recognize the humor that is evident in the average day of working with people and their animals.

I have enjoyed working in a large group practice after so many years of practicing alone. The new graduates really have a much better education than I, but I have the experience of having seen so much. I like working with younger people. We learn from each other.

We have so much more to work with today. The modern laboratory is one of the best things to happen to veterinary practice. We can do complete blood counts, blood chemistries, and bacteriology right here in the clinic. We used to have to guess and practice by the seat of our pants. Now we can really zero in on a diagnosis. The newer anesthetics are much safer for the animal, and modern radiology equipment is much safer for those of us who operate it. We can stay current with all the wonderful reference books that are available today. In the old days we had out-of-date books, often written by foreign authors.

The experience that I had, working before all the modern conveniences, is valuable too. I can offer alternatives to clients. Rather than euthanize an animal because its owner cannot afford diagnostic tests or expensive treatment or surgery, I may say, "This is the best method of ministering to your animal. However, we can try this alternative method for a minimal amount of money and see what response we get." Sometimes we surprise ourselves.

It is interesting to observe how veterinarians in other areas of the world do things. I have treated myself in recent years to some wonderful trips. I made a veterinary tour of China in 1983 with a group of nine veterinarians and spouses. I was somewhat shocked to find that there were no pet dogs or cats in China. It was all the people could do to feed themselves. They certainly couldn't feed pets. There was also the fear of rabies and toxoplasmosis.

The training of veterinarians in that country is far behind the training that we receive in the United States. We toured one of the veterinary schools in Inner Mongolia. We were especially interested in learning more about acupuncture, and I asked if we could have a demonstration. The dean, who was conducting our tour, asked an assistant to administer acupuncture anesthesia to a horse. The assistant did his bit with the acupuncture needles and then made an incision through the muscle of the horse. I was not impressed, because the poor beast jumped around like he could feel every cut and suture.

I also toured Australia with a group of veterinarians and their spouses in connection with the World Veterinary Congress in Perth. I roomed with Dr. Betty O'Connor, a veterinarian I had met on the China trip. When we reached Alice Springs, I decided that we should contact the local veterinarians. I called the only veterinary hospital in town, and we were all invited for a tour of Alice Springs Veterinary Hospital. The hospital was owned by a veterinary couple. These young veterinarians also provided the veterinary care for the racetrack and the rodeo. It just so happened that the second largest rodeo in Australia was in town, and our new friends invited our group to attend. It was a really wild rodeo, complete with aborigines and cowboys and much imbibing of beer and wine. The Country Race Meet was more sedate, but nevertheless we were advised to stay off the highway that evening.

I just recently returned from my second trip to Africa. This continent, with all its exotic animals and colorful people, has such an attraction for me. A friend and I spent two weeks on a safari to Kenya and Tanzania and then spent a week with my former employer, Dr. Vern Pedersen, and his wife, who now work as Peace Corps volunteers at the Mikolongwe Veterinary Station in Malawi.

Dr. Pedersen is the only veterinarian at the station and works with the local farmers. He does a lot of artificial insemination of cattle, trying to improve the quality of the herds, and oversees a large poultry-hatching operation. It ships about ten thousand hatching eggs a week to farmers all over Malawi.

The cattle operation there is quite interesting. The farmers are crossing cows of high-milk-producing breeds such as holstein-Friesians with Brahman bulls to produce a hardy crossbreed with natural disease resistance. However, the political system in Malawi is stripping the station of breeding bulls. The Malawi people just love the Brahmans because they are so big and striking with that hump on their back and the large droopy ears. The political officials come by and see the bulls and want to buy one or two to give as a gift to His Excellency, the lifetime president of Malawi, in return for political favors. It would be politically unwise for Dr. Pedersen to refuse to sell the bulls, so the station must continually import Brahman bulls while the presidential palace is probably overrun with them.

It was such a wonderful opportunity to be introduced to the people of that country by someone who lives and works there. We were invited into the homes and into the school and church. My traveling companion for the trip was a retired principal of an elementary school, and she was particularly interested in visiting a grade school.

Each grade is made up of approximately one hundred

children, all of whom sit on the floor. They had been expecting us, and when we arrived, they stood up and said in singsong English, "Good morning, Madam!"

My friend had brought school supplies such as paper, pencils, and yellow happy-face stickers, which were an instant hit. The schoolchildren have very little in the way of supplies, just a few notebooks in the upper grades, so our goodies were very useful to them. The people of Africa are very nice, really friendly, and so appreciative of everything.

I love to go to other countries, especially those that are considered underdeveloped in comparison with ours, and learn about the people, how they do things, and what they think. There is always a common bond between people from different parts of the world, and veterinary medicine has been the bond that has opened doors for me.

I know that my interest and involvement in veterinary medicine has kept me young and interested in life. And in spite of all those early predictions about women veterinarians wasting their education, I am still at it.

Veterinary medicine is a wonderful field for women. It does require, however, more than a love of animals. You must have a scientific, inquiring mind and love learning, because learning becomes a lifelong commitment. You must be willing to keep reading, going to courses and workshops, and exchanging ideas with others.

I think it's harder today for a young woman veterinarian to establish a business of her own and combine family and business, because of the investment in money and time that is necessary to make that business a success.

In our day, most veterinary practices were small, and equipment was modest. It didn't cost that much to get into practice, but you had years and years of building that business until it started making money. Today it costs so much to start a new practice that most new graduates must work for someone else. However, in general the financial rewards come sooner, the hours are better, and the life-style is a little less restrictive when working in a group practice. Working for someone else involves finding good competent child care and an employer who is understanding and flexible. As more women veterinarians move into the work force, solutions to these problems will be found.

I am content to work part-time now because it allows time to do some of the other things that are important to me. Outside of veterinary medicine, the thing that has been the biggest source of pleasure to me is music.

I enjoy listening to all types of music, except heavy metal, which, in my mind, should not be called music. I enjoy performing piano and organ music, which I do on a regular basis at the Lynden United Methodist Church. When not playing, I sing tenor in the choir. I have been the church music chairperson for a number of years, and in this capacity I am in charge of putting on an annual fund-raising pops concert. We started the pops concert when we were trying to raise funds to purchase a fifty-thousand-dollar organ, and we had so much fun that we've continued the project. The upcoming pops will be our seventh.

I have been a part of this community for so long that I can't see myself leaving or retiring somewhere else. There are always compatible people to do things and take trips with. I have my own built-in support group.

My future goals include continuing my world travels, if my health permits, and spending more time with my daughters and grandsons. My younger daughter lives in California and was just admitted to the California bar. My older daughter lives in Dallas with my two grandsons and is an owner-operator of a tractor-trailer rig (eighteen-wheeler), which is leased to a van line and used for hauling furniture throughout forty-eight states.

I suppose retirement is a reality I must face in the near future, but leaving this profession, which has been such an important part of my life for so many years, is not something that fills me with a great deal of anticipation. How many people in other professions can say that? Let's hear it for veterinary medicine! ■

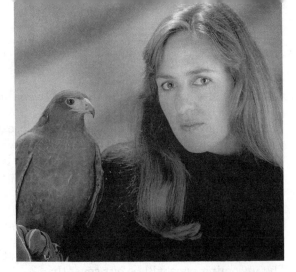

Susan K. Wells

BETWEEN New Orleans's Magazine Street and the Mississippi River sprawls the Audubon Park Zoo, one of the nation's ten top-rated zoos. Live oak trees dripping Spanish moss and the magenta blooms of giant azaleas in spring give living evidence that the grounds were once part of an old Louisiana plantation. The Audubon Park Zoo, as it exists today, is a quaint blending of the old with the new. The barn and stables, constructed in the 1930s, were renovated in 1980 to house the zoo's Animal Health Care Center.

It was also in 1980 that Susan K. Wells came to the Animal Health Care Center as a consulting veterinarian ministering to the zoo's creatures, great and small. Susan enjoyed working with exotic animals, and in 1985 she became the first full-time staff veterinarian at the zoo.

Wells's patients at Audubon represent three hundred different species and range in size from a three-gram hummingbird to a four-ton elephant. The large creatures like rhinoceros Jessie offer obvious challenges to the zoo's attending veterinarian. However, the small critters also require innovative means of observation, examination, and treatment.

The tiny hedgehog, a rodent that looks something like a prickly-pear cactus because of its porcupine-like quills, will curl into a spiked ball if approached. Wells says, "This little creature will fit in the palm of my hand. I can elect to examine him under anesthesia, but anesthetics can be risky in such small animals, as well as in the large ones. If I just want to take a quick peek at a lesion on a hedgehog's abdomen, I try to entice him to unroll and expose his soft underbelly. One way of doing this is to place the hedgehog in a plastic shoe box. Hopefully, when he feels it is safe to unwind, he will walk across the box and give me a quick view. It also works to place the animal on a plastic bread tray that has small holes in the surface. As the hedgehog walks along the tray surface, his legs fall through the holes, and I can examine him. The important thing about treating zoo animals is to create a safe and nonthreatening environment so they don't injure themselves or become distraught to the point that the medical problem is exacerbated."

Wells's job is more than coaxing a hedgehog to disarm its armor or a green sea turtle to stick its neck out of its shell. She also conducts research that will aid

244

in the understanding and care of zoo animals, and she educates others about the need to save our endangered animal and plant species.

Conservation of the world's natural resources is, in fact, Wells's crusade. A nonpretentious woman, Wells practices what she preaches. She and her husband, Chris, are vegetarians and advocates of recycling. Susan is an active member of Greenpeace, Defenders of Wildlife, World Wildlife Fund, the Nature Conservancy, and other organizations devoted to environmental issues.

Organizational veterinary medicine is another area in which Wells is making an impact for conservation. As 1989–90 president of the Association of Avian Veterinarians (AAV), an organization of more than two thousand practitioners involved in pet-bird medicine and in conservation, she is leading the entire profession to become stewards of the environment. The AAV board of directors recently voted unanimously to contribute 1 percent of the association's gross income to conservation projects, and Wells challenges other veterinary organizations to dedicate their resources in a similar manner to the preservation of the environment.

■

I have wonderful childhood memories of Sunday outings and birthday parties spent at the Lincoln Park Zoo in Chicago. When I first started dating my husband, Chris, we would meet at the polar bear exhibit at Lincoln Park. It was our favorite exhibit, and we knew all of the animals by name. Lincoln Park was important to me, just as Audubon Park occupies a place in the hearts of the people of New Orleans.

I am an only child, but I was surrounded by family when I was growing up. All of my aunts, uncles, and cousins lived in the same Chicago neighborhood. My father was employed by the postal department, and my mother worked as a waitress. When my mother first learned that I was accepted by the veterinary school, she cried. It wasn't that she didn't want me to become a veterinarian. She was upset because it meant that I would be moving away from Chicago and the family. My cousins, for the most part, stayed in the old neighborhood, living close to where they grew up. I am the only one who moved away.

I decided at an early age to become a veterinarian, because it was a way to combine both of my loves—animals and science. I grew up in the post-sputnik era, a time when schools really emphasized the space program and encouraged scientific endeavors.

In grade school, I designed numerous science projects, and I progressed until I won first prize at the Chicago Science Fair and then the Illinois State Science Fair.

After graduating from high school in 1969, I attended a commuter college, the Chicago Circle campus of the University of Illinois. After completing the preprofessional requirements, I applied to the veterinary school at the University of Illinois in Urbana. Much to my disappointment, I was turned down. At that time, there were six to seven applicants for each slot allotted to the freshman veterinary school class. My grade point average was competitive, but my scores on the veterinary school entrance exams were disappointing.

Perhaps everything happens for a reason. In an effort to improve my test scores, I decided to take the Stanley H. Kaplan course, which is designed to prepare students for medical career entrance tests. I was married to Chris by this time. We had met as teenagers at a muscular dystrophy camp in Michigan, where we were both counselors, and had married in 1970. I mentioned to the director of the Kaplan Center that my husband was looking for a job, and Chris's career with the Kaplan organization was thus conceived.

In the meantime, discouraged that I might not be accepted into veterinary school, I obtained a B.A. degree in sociology with a chemistry minor. The sociology courses were entertaining and rounded out my education, but veterinary medicine remained my goal. The Kaplan course really helped me improve my showing on the entrance tests, and I was accepted into the College of Veterinary Medicine at the University of Illinois in 1975.

Chris worked for the Kaplan organization during the four years that I was in veterinary school and did such an excellent job implementing the curriculum and helping other students to achieve their career goals that he was offered a promotion and transfer to New Orleans after I graduated from veterinary school.

During veterinary school, I set my sights on small-animal practice because zoo-animal medicine, my first choice, was discouraged. My instructors said, "There are few available jobs, and they are all political." Now that I am working in the field, I acknowledge the fact that jobs for veterinarians at zoos are limited compared with other specialties. However, I have not found politics to be a factor.

Even as late as the seventies, zoo medicine and wildlife medicine were in their inception. Few programs for training students existed, and few professors had the knowledge or experience to encourage students to pursue this area. One of my classmates who was interested in wildlife brought wild animals into the classroom and stimulated class participation. Today several veterinary schools have good training programs in exotic-animal medicine.

My husband's transfer to New Orleans coincided with my graduation, so I sent my résumé to a University of Illinois graduate who owned a large corporation of small-animal practices in New Orleans. I was hired over the telephone.

I worked at the St. Bernard Veterinary Hospital in Chalmette, a suburb of New Orleans. This clinic was one of eight outpatient clinics that were structured around a central hospital. The central-hospital concept had certain economic advantages because it allowed the corporation to order drugs and supplies in bulk and to share expensive equipment. The laboratory, radiographic equipment, and hospitalization facilities were located at the central hospital. Animals requiring those services were transported from an outpatient clinic to the central hospital by the pet owner or by hospital van.

I had worked at the St. Bernard Veterinary Hospital only six months when the owner was killed in an automobile accident. After the organization was restructured, I began working at the Algiers Animal Hospital. Old Junius, an elderly Cajun gentleman, came with the Algiers hospital. I was the only woman veterinarian in the corporation at that time, and I think Junius was fascinated by a woman doctor. Junius had never been to school, but he had worked with and treated animals for years. He had many old formulas, but he would never reveal the secret ingredients to any of the rest of us. The amazing thing was that some of Junius's remedies worked quite well. For example, a coughing dog would come in, and Junius would mix up a homemade cough syrup for it. Most of the time, the dog stopped coughing. Although his methods could hardly be considered modern sophisticated veterinary medicine, Junius taught me how to improvise.

The move to the Algiers hospital also brought the opportunity to work with Dr. Andy Gutter, the consulting veterinarian for the Audubon Park Zoo and the man who became my mentor in zoo-animal medicine. I had only been at the hospital a few days when I approached Dr. Gutter about working with him at the zoo. Dr. Gutter told me, "We'll both go to the zoo a couple of mornings each week for a month, and then you can go on your own."

Dr. Gutter and I had visited the zoo only two or three times when he was invited to travel to Kenya. He provided me with telephone numbers for five experienced zoo veterinarians whom I could call if I needed advice while he was in Africa, and then he left me in charge. His instructions were "Just don't kill the gorilla!"

I had been out of veterinary school about six months, and having full responsibility for the zoo animals was intimidating. However, nothing terrible happened while Dr. Gutter was away, and being forced into a situation of responsibility without having someone looking over your shoulder can be a great learning tool. I find myself using that tactic with veterinary students who spend their preceptorships here. You really find out quickly what you can do, and it builds confidence.

I learned a lot about zoo medicine from Dr. Gutter. He had worked at the Brookfield Zoo in Chicago and treated exotic animals in private practice. He and I shared the zoo work until 1985 when I become the full-time staff veterinarian at Audubon Park. Dr. Gutter is currently a consultant to the zoo, and we recently hired a second veterinarian to share responsibilities at the zoo and the Aquarium of the Americas, which opened in the French Quarter in September 1990.

The different species of aquatic animals that are displayed at the aquarium provide new diagnostic challenges for me, but that's part of what keeps my job interesting. I feel fortunate that I had five years of small-animal practice experience prior to working full-time at the zoo. Procedures like eye enucleations and cesarean sections, which are routine in veterinary practice, are occasionally performed on zoo animals too. It is helpful that I've had experience working with dogs and cats that I can apply to the variety of species I now work with.

The reason that people work in the zoo setting is to make a contribution to animals. Zoo work is a labor of love. Most of us, from the keepers on up to the administrators, could double our salaries in industry. We have several keepers who have advanced college degrees. I accepted a substantial pay cut when I left practice and became a full-time employee of the zoo.

I work with physicians and veterinarians who generously donate their expertise, time, and equipment to help our animals. For example, we took one of the monkeys to a local medical facility for an echocardiology evaluation of a heart murmur. Dr. Bob Beckerman, a faculty member at Tulane Medical Center, is a pediatrician who serves as a consultant for our great ape babies, and other specialists are available if we need them. The professionals who volunteer their services seem to have fun and enjoy the novelty of working with different species, and their expertise allows us to provide better care for the animals.

People sometimes think veterinarians would rather be M.D.'s, but I have not found this to be the case. In fact, I recently talked to a physician who is considering applying to veterinary school because he really wants to be a veterinarian.

The Audubon zoo includes the Wild Bird Rehabilitation Center, which provides medical and supportive care for birds that have been injured or orphaned. The rehab center was started initially by one of the keepers who lived on the zoo grounds. The injured birds needing assistance soon outgrew her small apartment. Now the rehab center harbors approximately eighteen hundred birds a year and has two full-time staff members devoted to its operation.

Zoo medicine is very much a cooperative endeavor. I depend upon the keepers to bring problems to my attention. They are the ones who have intimate daily contact with the animals and notice subtle changes with their charges.

Preventative medicine is very important in a zoo setting. Animals are examined routinely and, if necessary, vaccinated against infectious diseases. Newly arrived animals must pass three negative tests for parasites before they leave quarantine to be placed in an exhibit. Because of our hot and humid climate, parasites such as hookworms are a year-round problem.

Wild animals can often be ill without manifesting clinical signs of disease. Nature has provided them with an amazing ability to mask symptoms of illness or injury because, in the wild, the sick and weak fall victim to predators.

There is more judgment involved in treating zoo animals than in treating domestic pets. I have to make the decision that the diagnostic information or treatment is worth the risk of restraint or anesthesia before I proceed. Our animals are hard to replace, and certain animals such as the gorillas are beyond price.

Several years ago, we immobilized Rosebud the hippopotamus to implant a birth-control device. If she had fallen incorrectly, she could have been severely injured. It took all of us, including keepers, curators, and veterinary technicians, for that procedure.

We recently anesthetized Jessie, one of the rhinoceroses, for diagnostic testing after preliminary tests suggested tuberculosis. I performed a TB test and drew blood for laboratory testing, while veterinarians from the veterinary school of Louisiana State University at Baton Rouge performed a bronchoscopic exam. Luckily, the tests were all negative for TB.

Most of the larger animals, like Rosebud and Jessie, must be anesthetized before examination or treatment. Animals such as the zebras are impossible to handle for hoof trimming or other routine husbandry procedures if they are not immobilized first.

Working with M99, a drug used primarily to immobilize hoofstock, is perhaps one of the most dangerous aspects of my job. It is a wonderful drug and can be reversed by an intravenous antidote. However, the lethal dose of this drug for humans is a fraction of a milliliter. A veterinarian in England died when he accidentally injected himself with M99. We are very careful, and I have written emergency protocols to prevent accidents.

My job is not just working with animals. I have administrative duties, such as developing the budget, and I supervise the staffs of both the commissary and the hospital. The commissary is devoted to the dietary care of the entire collection of approximately sixteen hundred animals. The hospital staff consists of two veterinary technicians who care for hospitalized and quarantined animals. I also take on the role of educator and researcher.

One of my research projects involves monitoring the reproductive cycles of our elephants. We take blood samples weekly and measure the progesterone hormone levels. This information will help us develop a reproductive program for Asian elephants, which are an endangered species.

I am the primary investigator at Audubon Park working with an Institute of Museum Services grant to develop a medical management manual for orangutans. The orangutan is one of twenty-six species managed under a species survival plan (SSP). The SSP program, which is under the direction of the American Association of Zoological Parks and Aquariums, is a cooperative effort intended to insure the long-term survival and genetic diversity of critical species. Zoos participating in this program share knowledge and animals.

My associates, Eva Sargent, Ph.D., and Mark Andrews, were instrumental in assisting me with the SSP project. The finished product covers computerization of medical records, as well as medical disorders of orangutans. We hope that the techniques we have developed will serve as a model for evaluation of medical problems in other SSP species.

Public relations is a fun part of my job. If we have an

unusual surgery or interesting case, it is covered by newspapers, radio, and television. My greatest claim to fame was when I was featured on the "Captain Kangaroo" TV show several years ago. The television crew filmed several short segments that showed me performing physical examinations on an elephant and a litter of fox babies. A friend from college whom I hadn't communicated with in fifteen years called after her children spotted me on "Captain Kangaroo." Several veterinary school classmates telephoned after seeing my picture on the monthly Purina calendar, which was mailed to veterinary offices across the country.

The media work and the zoo-sponsored seminars I present are great vehicles for educating the public about the zoo and about ecology. My role as a teacher is sometimes direct and sometimes indirect. I directly supervise veterinary students from various schools who elect to spend a six-week zoo-medicine preceptorship with us, and I indirectly assist my colleagues at Central American zoos.

During the summer of 1988 I attended the first Central American Symposium on the Administration and Management of Zoological Parks, in Guatemala City, Guatemala. I found that the zoos in Central and South America are not as developed as ours in terms of facilities or resources, but that doesn't seem to affect their visitation. The number of people who visit and enjoy these zoos is phenomenal, and zoo personnel are in an excellent position to communicate with the local residents about their unique resources of plants and animals.

The symposium was a great place to exchange ideas and meet the people who support and work at Central American zoos. We are now trying to set up a networking system with our colleagues there. A veterinarian from Costa Rica will soon be spending a couple of months at Audubon Park Zoo helping develop a program for the training of foreign veterinarians.

I also participate in the Zoo Conservation Outreach Group, a team of twenty-five U.S. zoos dedicated to assisting Central American zoos and their local conservation efforts. The Audubon Park Zoo will serve as a clearinghouse for used veterinary texts and journals, which will be donated to La Aurora Zoo in Guatemala City. La Aurora Zoo will house a central reference library and distribute scientific literature to other Central American zoos.

I am the cochairperson of a one-day session on animals of tropical America that will be part of the 1990 Conference of the American Association of Zoo Veterinarians. We are currently soliciting funds to assist our Central and South American colleagues with conference expenses and to provide bilingual translation of the entire five-day meeting.

Half of the world's tropical rain forests are located in Central and South America. Rain forests cover only 6 percent of the earth but provide homes for 50 percent of all animal species. Tropical rain forests are being destroyed in favor of logging, cattle grazing, and agriculture. As the land is cleared, more and more species vanish. The richness of the rain forests is in the biological cycles that take place in the canopies. The soil is actually very poor, and the cleared land becomes a desert after a few years of use. At least twenty-seven million acres of rain forest—an area the size of Pennsylvania—are destroyed each year. The world's critical mass of rain forests may be gone by the year 2000, and with it will go our global climate as we know it.

Africa is another area with dwindling natural resources. Elephants, rhinoceroses, and mountain gorillas could disappear in our lifetime. The issues there are immensely complex. A native poacher on a subsistence living can feed a family for two years with money received from a poached rhino. We are not going to solve animal problems as long as there are starving humans in an area. The people who live in countries with wildlife resources must feel it is in their best interest to preserve them. The tourist trade may prove to be that reason. Photography tours are replacing many of the big-game safaris. Tourists need hotels and restaurants, and this creates jobs.

In Zimbabwe, new tribal programs allow hunting expeditions. They permit a controlled number of animals to be killed. Since these projects began, illegal poaching has been reduced by 90 percent in some areas. I'm not for trophy hunting. However, we may have to make this kind of compromise to save endangered animals from extinction. With poaching under control, enough animals are left to breed and sustain the species.

The people in the United States are the largest consumers of wildlife in the world. We import more than $600 million worth of wildlife and wildlife products each year. The education of the U.S. public is one of the keys to changing this situation.

I emphasize conservation when I talk to zoo and civic groups. I inform people about our endangered species and the destruction of critical wildlife habitats. I discourage them from buying wild animal products, such as ivory, and from keeping exotic animals as pets.

Lions and other wild animals cannot be properly housed

and cared for by pet owners. I have seen cases of monkeys that have had their teeth pulled so they will be less of a danger to their human owners. These animals become social misfits. They cannot be integrated back with animals of their own kind, and it's a cruel injustice.

I think that we can do much to preserve our environment if we will just be aware and evaluate how we live our individual lives. We can choose products that are biodegradable and produced by companies that support environmental issues. Consumer guides are available that rate companies in such categories as animal testing and environmental protection. We can write to company presidents and politicians about our concerns for the environment. We can also join groups such as the World Wildlife Fund, Greenpeace, and the Nature Conservancy.

Our zoo has become more conservation-conscious, and we try to set an example for the community. We have located newspaper bins in convenient places so people can drive by and donate their old newspapers. We are recycling cans, glass, and plastic too. The recycling project has made several thousand dollars, which we dedicate to outside conservation projects. One year the money was donated to the World Wildlife Fund, and it was earmarked for the restoration of rain forests in Costa Rica. We thought this was an appropriate use of the money because trees are used to make paper products, and we were sending money back to support the rain forests where trees had been cut down.

Conservation issues are now being addressed in the media, and people are thinking about them. New biodegradable products are showing up in the marketplace. I am much more optimistic about the future of the environment because of this increased awareness.

Veterinarians are in a unique position to educate the public about the need to preserve animals and the environment. At a recent board meeting of the Association of Avian Veterinarians (AAV), we voted to dedicate 1 percent of our gross income to conservation, and as president, I have sent a letter to all the state and specialty veterinary organizations, urging them to consider a similar commitment. If every organization and every individual donated 1 percent, it would make a significant contribution toward saving our planet.

The Association of Avian Veterinarians is made up primarily of practitioners. These are people who own their own practices, and we run the AAV as a successful nonprofit organization. We offer scholarships for externships in avian medicine to qualified senior veterinary students, fund research projects pertaining to captive-bird health, and educate the public about pet birds.

The majority of birds are captured in the wild because domestic breeding can't keep up with the demand. Approximately 800,000 birds, one-third of them parrots, are imported into the United States each year. We could easily deplete the wild population of many species.

Most people don't realize where their birds come from. A tree in the rain forest is hacked down, and the mother bird may be killed so that her babies can be sold to a pet store in the United States. The young birds, which are already severely stressed, spend a month in government quarantine before they even get to that pet store. At least a third of these birds die before they reach the owner's home.

In border areas of the United States, bird smuggling is big business. A South American macaw, which costs only a few dollars to capture, may sell for fifteen hundred dollars or more in a pet store. This kind of profit margin makes heavy losses acceptable to the importer. Smuggled birds, which bypass quarantine, often die of disease and stress or pass infections to other birds or owners.

I am not trying to discourage people from owning pet birds, because they make wonderful companion animals. However, I feel that pet ownership is a responsibility, and potential owners should think about what is going on in the pet-bird industry. I hope more people will make sure that the bird they are purchasing is domestically raised rather than wild-caught. Domestically raised birds are better choices because they are generally more healthy and make better pets than those brought in from the wild.

My husband, Chris, and I adopted two birds. The cockatiel, Yaeger, fell from the sky into my neighbor's yard one Thanksgiving, and we adopted him. The parrot is a recycled pet, which was donated to the zoo about ten years ago by an owner who was tired of it.

Our other pets include three cats, two dogs, and a horse. The horse represents the fulfillment of an adolescent dream. I have little free time, but I try to ride him once or twice a week. Our fourteen-year-old dog was rescued from the pharmacology lab when I was a veterinary student. We just recently lost our oldest cat, which had also joined us after a few close encounters in a research lab.

Chris and I have been together more than twenty years and share many of the same ideas and interests. We decided to become vegetarians because that is one more choice we can make toward conservation. We are both students of karate and highly recommend it to others.

Martial arts training teaches you to be humble, both mentally and physically. I have learned to focus my attention better and be present in the moment. These skills are helpful in my work. My reaction time is quicker, which is important when I am working with zoo animals and the immobilizing drug M99.

My husband is very supportive of my career. When we first married in the sixties, we bought into the American dream and planned to have seven strong sons. When I pursued my own dream of working as a veterinarian, children became less of a priority. My career takes a lot of energy. I feel it would be a sacrifice to have children and do it right, and I sure wouldn't want to do it wrong.

Chris and I led a group of eighteen people on a trip to Kenya in 1986 as part of the Audubon Park Zoo's travel program. It was a thrill to see animal species that I work with every day in their natural habitats. We tried to make the trip interesting for the participants with anecdotes about my experiences with some of the species we observed.

When Chris and I take vacations, we prioritize the countries we would like to visit. We go first to those places with resources of animals and natural beauty that might disappear in our lifetime. We recently visited Costa Rica and Guatemala.

Someday we would like to do a field project. The Morris Animal Foundation established an animal hospital in Rawanda, Africa, shortly after Dian Fossey's death. The foundation accepts selected veterinarians for a period of six months to one year. Veterinarians participate in research and monitor the health of the same gorilla population that Fossey studied. I would like to have this type of experience.

It is through studies like Fossey's that we have learned vital information about the nature of animal behavior in the wild. Modern zoos have incorporated that knowledge into the design of facilities and the care and handling of the animals. The early zoos had postage-stamp collections, with one monkey in a cage next to another monkey in a cage. Monkeys don't live like that in the wild. They live in family groups.

The Audubon Park Zoo, now a part of the Audubon Institute, has done a lot to update and renovate existing facilities. The city of New Orleans passed three major bond issues in the seventies to fund most of this work. Three years ago the city passed a bond issue to fund the Aquarium of the Americas, which will be a wonderful addition to the riverfront area. People who grew up in New Orleans have seen the changes and have confidence and pride in what can be done here to preserve animals and nature. Ron Forman, our zoo director, is a dynamic individual and is the driving force behind these projects.

Patrons of the zoo often take an interest in individual animals. When Rosebud the hippopotamus died, people came to her exhibit and left flowers, sympathy cards, and notes. It seemed to me that people wanted to personally acknowledge their grief for the passing of an animal they had appreciated and loved.

People like to be intimately involved. One of the zoo's fund-raising projects is the Adopt an Animal Program. An individual can sponsor a Madagascar cockroach for fifteen dollars a year or an orangutan for a larger amount of money. People feel that they have a personal relationship with the animal they adopt. They can say, "I helped feed Frankie the orangutan." Plus, projects like this significantly help the zoo finance day-to-day operations.

Audubon Park has made an effort to display and preserve the flora and fauna indigenous to this area of south Louisiana. Five of the live oak trees are listed by the Live Oak Society because of their longevity. The Louisiana Swamp display presents a microcosm of the wildlife, plants, and people who have lived in this environment for centuries.

I am proud of the zoo and enjoy veterinary medicine and my job as zoo veterinarian. The challenges are still stimulating to me. I accept the sometimes mundane administrative chores because I know that I have an opportunity to contribute to the preservation of animals and our environment. Zoos are wonderful vehicles for teaching stewardship of the planet. This is satisfying work. ∎

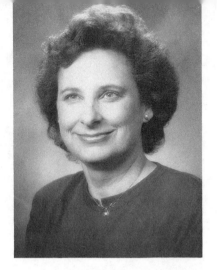

H. Ellen Whiteley

AS some people mingle entrees on a plate, H. Ellen Whiteley mixes the talents and tools of her trades—veterinary medicine and writing—in a small office behind her home. The cold shiny surfaces of stainless steel—cages, surgery table, sterilizer—coexist with the beige plastic of a computer, a printer, and a word processor. The back-and-forth whine of the printer sometimes muffles the protests of her feline patients, but the hospital odors—alcohol and disinfectant—easily snuff out the faint emanation of printing ink and pencil lead.

Whiteley is the owner-operator of Cat Clinic of Amarillo, which is a house-call service for cats in Amarillo, Texas, and Professional Veterinary Services, a free-lance writing business. A veterinarian with twenty-two years of experience, Whiteley says she has made good progress toward experiencing every facet of veterinary medicine. She has trained with the U.S. Department of Agriculture, worked as a staff veterinarian for a state department of agriculture, worked in industry—both as a laboratory-animal veterinarian and in marketing—served as an Army Reserve veterinarian, directed and taught a veterinary technology program, and practiced small-animal medicine in four states.

A woman who likes change and challenge, Whiteley knows that a twenty-year retirement pin is not in her future. "I am fortunate," she says, "that veterinary medicine offers great opportunities for me to see, be, and do different things. Most of my professional endeavors have enhanced my abilities to perform the others." She utilized her practice skills when she served as base veterinarian for the military, her laboratory-animal knowledge when treating a pet rabbit, her marketing know-how when designing the Cat Clinic brochure, her regulatory insight when working for industry, and everything when teaching.

Whiteley's veterinary experience and credentials have opened doors for her in the publishing industry. She has written pet- and veterinary-related columns appearing in the *Saturday Evening Post, Woman's World,* the *Milwaukee Sentinel,* the *Amarillo Daily News,* and *dvm,* as well as articles for consumer and professional magazines. Her article "Animals Are Good for What Ails You," published in the *Saturday*

Evening Post, won the 1985 National Media Award presented by the Delta Society.

Whiteley's talent as communicator in the spoken word gives her the opportunity for travel and adventure. As a panel member of the Purina Pet Parent Program, she journeyed to New York City to join actor and spokesperson Alan Thicke and the press at the 21 Club. She flew to Ely, Minnesota, with two other writers to interview antarctic explorer Will Steger and sampled the rigors of sled-dog travel firsthand. She has appeared on more than one hundred radio and television programs and has spoken to state and local audiences, including the Delaware Senate, to veterinarians attending the Pennsylvania annual conference, and to physicians at the Texas Tech University Health Sciences Center.

Whiteley was chosen for inclusion in the 1987–88 first edition of *Who's Who in Veterinary Science and Medicine.* She is married, the mother of four children, and a coauthor of this book.

∎

The first initial in my name stands for "Henry." Although I've tried in later years to circumvent problems by using a first initial, I've found that the monicker at times had its advantages, as well as disadvantages.

Way back, when girls did not belong to the Future Farmers of America (FFA), I did. With a name like Henry, no one was the wiser until our high school chapter traveled out of town. I was the only female to make the illustrious bus trip to Baton Rouge, Louisiana, for the state livestock show and rodeo. And then the rodeo tried to refuse me admission on my FFA identification. On my eighteenth birthday, I received a notice from the local draft board. I'm sure the board thought that some individuals would do anything to avoid being one of a "few good men" when I wrote back to inform the board that I was female.

But I've always tried to look on the bright side. My mother opted to name me Henry Ellen after my grandfather and grandmother rather than John Henry after my father and grandfather.

I grew up in a small house adjacent to my grandparents' larger house in Jonesville, Louisiana. When I was ten years old, my family—which included my mother, stepfather, and younger brother, Joel—moved to a dairy farm on the outskirts of town. I took to rural life like the proverbial duck to water. When other girls my age were taking ballet and piano lessons or playing in the band, I was building fences and a barn for my jersey 4-H calves. Joel summed up my aspirations quite aptly when he said, "My sister is agricultural, not cultural."

My mother, who tended to be a cynic, was fond of saying that animals and children were miserable little creatures. This sentiment didn't keep me from playing nursemaid to a variety of animals, including dogs, hogs, bantam chickens, polled Hereford bulls, and jersey heifers. However, I will admit that there have been times in my own nurturing career that I've agreed with Mother's viewpoint about the children.

My family expected me to be responsible, work hard, and become a professional woman. Marriage and family were never expressed as priorities. I have read that the firstborn child tries to fulfill the aspirations of the father. I think my stepfather might have pursued veterinary medicine if circumstances had permitted. When I attended Louisiana State University in Baton Rouge in 1962, he sold the dairy and went to college with me to seek a degree in animal science.

My preprofessional advisers at LSU tried to discourage me from choosing veterinary medicine as a career. Louisiana did not have a veterinary school at that time and sent only a limited number of students each year to veterinary schools at Auburn, Oklahoma State, and Texas A&M universities. The sentiment was this: "We sent Miss X and she flunked out, and then Miss V got married in veterinary school and dropped out. We can't waste our few veterinary slots on females who won't finish."

Obviously, I made it to veterinary school. Much credit goes to my reluctant male mentors who saw my determination and rewarded and encouraged me with a summer job at the LSU veterinary science department and with scholarships. At the end of two years at LSU, I applied to veterinary schools at Texas A&M University and Oklahoma State University in Stillwater.

I received a letter of acceptance and a document from Texas A&M detailing conduct considered appropriate for professional women. Professional concerns included warnings about student marriage and a statement that the professional woman does not wear jewelry. I am sure that accepting women in that traditional male university setting was very worrisome to those used to the status quo. I was to be in the second veterinary class open to women; the class before had one woman, Sonja Oliphant Lee. When I received a letter of acceptance from Oklahoma State University, I decided to go to Oklahoma.

I remember my first day at veterinary school. I couldn't find the room where the veterinary school dean was scheduled to present "Orientation and Remarks," and I was too bashful to ask anyone. I passed a man, leaning against the door frame in the hall, who remarked, "Another goddamn woman." I thought he was joking, but he wasn't. He turned out to be one of my professors.

There were four women and forty-four men in my freshman class. The sophomore class had no women. I tried to hide in the back of the room that first semester, but it was impossible to remain unobtrusive. The first months were hard, and all of us, male and female, were scared that we didn't have what it took to make it.

I found my classmates to be friendly, although some with tact and others with less tact expressed the opinion that we four women were holding veterinary school slots that could have gone to men and that we would just get married and have babies and waste our education. The three of us who graduated are all still working as veterinarians. We also married and had children.

I remember the ambiguity of my feelings toward my male classmates. Because I was from out of state and knew few people outside of veterinary school, I wanted very much to fit in and belong. The class was a close group, studying together and drinking beer together after tests. I found myself walking a fine line between maintaining my femininity and being one of the boys.

There were advantages and disadvantages for women in veterinary school at that time. It was harder because of the uncertainty of our roles and because we were constantly put in a position of proving ourselves. If a woman veterinary student was too aggressive and masculine, she was perceived as a woman who wanted to be a man. If she was too pretty and feminine, she was suspected of being there to catch a man. On the other hand, we were different and stood out from the crowd. Being the first has its own rewards.

At the start of my last semester at veterinary school, I married Gary White, a classmate, and at graduation became Dr. Henry Ellen Rayl White. Many marriages occur among students in veterinary school. Students work and study and play in such proximity that romance often blossoms. However, I dated veterinary students who told me that our relationship would never be serious, because they didn't want a wife who was a professional equal. Those were the days when many men desired a wife who would look up to them. I think that most men today prefer a wife who will help share the load.

After graduation, my husband entered the Army and served a tour of duty in Vietnam. During that time, I trained with the U.S. Department of Agriculture's Poultry Inspection Service in Minnesota. When my daughter Susan was born, I retired from poultry inspection before assuming a permanent position.

After my husband returned from Vietnam, we worked for a brief period in a small-animal practice in Dallas. Then Gary became disenchanted with our employer, and we moved to New Orleans so he could pursue a residency program in laboratory-animal medicine at Tulane University.

In New Orleans, I visited several veterinary hospitals to solicit employment as a small-animal practitioner. An older veterinarian made this comment: "Well, honey, I can't hire you, but I sure can use your husband." Another time, a practitioner who had hired me for a week of relief work called to cancel at the last minute. I learned later that he believed the rumor that I was not really licensed but was practicing under my husband's license. I eventually found jobs with veterinarians who believed I could do the work, but for the most part, older practitioners found it hard to accept women as real veterinarians because we were so new. A woman who had graduated from Texas A&M and I were the first two women to be licensed to practice in the state of Louisiana. That was in 1970.

I spent my first twelve years as a veterinarian practicing small-animal medicine in three different states. As the years passed, I noticed a change in the way women clients related to me as a veterinarian. During the early years when I worked with male colleagues, the clients, predominantly women, seemed to prefer the men I worked with, especially if the men happened to be good communicators or handsome. Then came a time when I thought I had the advantage. I matured and became more confident, but women in general became more supportive of each other. When I opened my practice in Edmond, Oklahoma, in 1979, female pet owners seemed to seek me out.

Clients began to express the opinion that women veterinarians were more gentle with their pets. Women with small children often felt more at ease with me because I had children of my own and catered to the young people who came in my practice by setting up a special children's area in the waiting room, complete with puzzles, books, and coloring books about animals.

The major responsibility for caring for my own children fell on me. My second daughter, Kimberly, was born in 1974, and during the years when my daughters were young, I felt torn in many directions. When the children were sick and could not go to day care or to school, they went with me to a veterinary hospital. When it was my own hospital, it was a good solution. When I worked for someone else, it was a questionable decision. I often carried a sleeping toddler with me to a clinic for a late-night or early-morning emergency call. Other times, I responded to late-night emergencies by sneaking out of the house while the girls stayed at home in bed. If they accompanied me, I felt guilty about keeping the older one up on a school night, and if I left them at home, I felt guilty too.

After my husband had completed his lab-animal residency, we practiced together for a period of time. Veterinary medicine seemed to be the glue that held our marriage together. We talked about cases at home, clients accepted us as interchangeable Siamese twins, and I had a partner with the confidence to perform my difficult orthopedic surgeries. When the marriage ended, I was devastated. Later I realized that it was the best thing that could have happened to me. As a single woman, I was forced to make decisions about cases, perform my own surgery, and most of all, take responsibility for my personal and professional choices.

After the divorce, I decided to leave Oklahoma and start new somewhere else. I put my small-animal practice up for sale and began applying for out-of-state nonpractice jobs. During this time, I received a telephone call from an Army recruiter. She asked, "Are you the Dr. White who is inquiring about the Army?"

I laughed because joining the military had never entered my mind. However, the more I thought about it, the more I liked the idea. I went for my physical and filled out what seemed like a million government forms. I thought that my application was just a formality. I had veterinary experience, good grades in college, licenses to practice veterinary medicine in three states, and letters of recommendation that made me look as if I could almost walk on water. Then the shock came—the Army turned me down.

I was told that because of my years of experience I would qualify to enter the Veterinary Corps as a major, a rank above many experienced veterinary officers who were only captains, and that the Army didn't want to condone such a situation. I was very disappointed and volunteered to start at the same rank as everyone else. I was told that my rank was dictated by law.

I tried once more. I asked the colonel with whom I was pleading if it made any difference that I was the daughter of a veteran killed in World War II. He replied, "It holds more weight that you were the wife of a veterinary officer who served in

Vietnam, but that won't get you in either."

Although I wasn't able to run off and join the Army or the circus, a miracle occurred. A young woman who had recently graduated from veterinary school at Oklahoma State decided to buy my clinic at the same time that I was offered a job with the Oklahoma Department of Agriculture in Oklahoma City. Although Oklahoma City wasn't as far away as I had hoped to travel, I decided to take the job.

Selling Downtown Animal Clinic was somewhat like selling one of the children. I had designed the interior, chosen the colors and equipment, and practiced my way for the first time in my life. However, I liked the veterinarian who bought the clinic, and I felt good about leaving it with her.

I was apprehensive about my qualifications as a staff veterinarian for the Oklahoma Department of Agriculture because of my inexperience in large-animal production and medicine. State veterinarians work primarily to control animal diseases harmful to the state's agricultural industry. I told the veterinarian who interviewed me that except for veterinary school, I had had no significant large-animal experience since leaving the farm when I was seventeen years old. He replied, "But you speak the language and understand rural people."

I immediately called my brother and told him that the fact that I was agricultural instead of cultural had finally paid off. I stayed with the department for only five months, but I learned to respect regulatory veterinarians and the work they perform.

I had continued to send out résumés for nonpractice jobs located at least five hundred miles from Oklahoma. It wasn't that I disliked Oklahoma or veterinary practice. I just felt the intense desire to start over in a new location with a different professional challenge. I applied for numerous jobs for which I had no experience, and I finally decided that I wasn't qualified to do anything except practice small-animal medicine. About the time I was ready to give up, I talked to a veterinarian about a job in the veterinary pharmaceutical industry. I lamented about trying to change professional directions after twelve years in practice. He said, "You are doing the right thing. I firmly believe in changing careers at least every ten years because the new challenges keep you fresh and excited about life."

My optimistic colleague inspired me to continue my job search, and I was finally offered a position as quality assurance veterinarian with Fromm Laboratories, an animal-vaccine company in Grafton, Wisconsin.

My job as quality assurance veterinarian required laboratory-animal medicine knowledge. Although I had no formal training in this discipline, I could, again, speak the language. Twelve years of marriage to a lab-animal veterinarian was on-the-job training of sorts. I supervised the testing of the company's vaccines in laboratory animals.

After two years in quality assurance, I moved to the marketing department to become the Fromm Laboratories rabies awareness spokesperson, a job that I still consider the opportunity of a lifetime. I worked closely with a public relations firm that represented Fromm. The public relations people hired a local television personality to teach me how to dress, apply makeup, and conduct myself on television. It was this country girl's first exposure to glamour and media hyperbole, and I loved it.

I traveled extensively, from California to New York, to appear on television and radio programs in an effort to alert the general public about the need for rabies prevention. I also wrote technical literature and communicated with veterinarians from all over the country. This job provided many professional perquisites but made my role as a single parent more difficult.

During this time, I decided to fulfill my earlier aspiration to join the military by becoming a member of the Wisconsin National Guard. The Army colonel had been correct—I entered the service at the rank of major. I became a member of a medical company—a unit of medics, physicians, nurses, and one veterinarian, me.

In many ways the Guard was my middle-age escapade. I learned to fire an M-16 rifle and .45 automatic, drive a deuce-and-a-half truck, and survive the litter obstacle course. It was exciting but was also one more obligation for which I had to scrounge time and energy.

Rather than accept the fact that life is sometimes better served by fewer accomplishments done well, I proceeded like a runaway train. I started an after-hours small-animal house-call service out of my home. In my spare time, after work and chauffeuring kids to ballet and soccer practice, I would drive to a client's home to treat a dog with a sore throat or give a rabies vaccination to a pet cat.

This was also the time when I got my first writing break. The *Milwaukee Sentinel* decided to publish "My First Case," the story of a severely injured kitten and my trepidations as a new veterinarian. I had written the story several years earlier and had spent an enormous amount of time polishing and rewriting it. In spite of all my hopes for the article, it had been rejected by what seemed like thousands of magazines. When I arrived in Wisconsin, I found "My First Case" as I was unpacking the moving boxes and sent it out one last time, to the *Sentinel*. On the basis of that article, the *Sentinel* gave me a column titled "Pets and People," which was published with my byline every few weeks in the Good Morning section of the paper. This story of my first experiences as a veterinarian was eventually published in an altered form in my *Saturday Evening Post* column, "Vets on Pets," which I started writing a short time later. Today, when I speak to writing groups, I always mention "My First Case" because it is an example of what it takes to succeed in the writing business—the confidence to persevere in the face of rejection.

In spite of my new opportunities in writing and practice, I knew that I couldn't continue all my professional obligations, because it wasn't fair to the children. But I enjoyed all of them—my full-time job at Fromm, the Guard, House Calls for Small Animals, and my columns in the *Sentinel* and the *Saturday Evening Post*. To give up any of them seemed like a sacrifice. Then the decision was taken out of my hands. The marketing department at Fromm Laboratories was transferred from the Grafton location to the parent company in Charles City, Iowa.

The girls and I had lived in Wisconsin for three years at this point and loved Cedarburg, the small picturesque community where we lived, and its wonderful people with ethnic names like "Burmeister" and "Cechlinski." We didn't want to move to a small town in Iowa. I contemplated staying in Cedarburg and developing House Calls, but I finally decided to give up everything and start over again with a new job in a new area of the country.

The girls and I moved one thousand miles, to Amarillo, Texas, where I accepted the position of coordinator of a new program of veterinary technology (VT) at Amarillo College. I had only worked a couple of weeks when I realized that I had tackled an overwhelming task.

The VT program is a two-year course of study designed to teach people to be veterinary assistants. The veterinary assistant is similar to a physician's assistant. He or she is trained to take medical histories and interact with veterinary clients, give medications, administer anesthesia, prepare animals for surgery, and perform laboratory and radiological procedures. These tasks assist large- and small-animal practitioners or veterinarians employed in other career fields such as zoos, industry, the military, or research.

I had worked with a couple of graduate veterinary technicians at Fromm Laboratories, but that was the extent of my experience in this relatively new field. I had never visited another VT program, and I had no idea of the hurdles ahead of me.

Those hurdles became real my first day on the job. Without having so much as one textbook or piece of equipment, any designated laboratory or animal space, or any program-owned animals, I started enrolling students for the fall semester. Within weeks, I was teaching, among other things, anatomy and physiology, a course that I hadn't even thought about for more than twenty years.

Students enrolled, so all I could do was to run with the ball. It didn't get any easier. At the end of two years, I was still struggling along without facilities or an additional instructor. The Texas economy was in the doldrums, which caused the college administrators to become even more reluctant to spend money to develop the program. Several times during the first two years, the administration toyed with the idea of dropping the program. I felt like I had been hired under false pretenses, and after three years, I resigned.

Although I suffered from immense feelings of self-doubt during my time at Amarillo College, I also made wonderful friends among the faculty and students. My rewards came from seeing students grow in self-esteem and knowledge. And perhaps knowledge was the lesser in importance of those two qualities. Most students in VT programs, including those receiving military training, are female. Many of these women are middle-aged, with family responsibilities, and are apprehensive about going back to college. Yet maturity counts for a whole lot, and most blossom into excellent students.

It has been said that veterinary technology is a woman's field because of low salaries for graduates. I believe that many men are turned off by the low starting wages, and when I directed the VT Program at Amarillo College, I wrestled with the fact that most of my graduates would start work at five dollars an hour.

However, the VT degree is a viable option for people who enjoy this kind of work but cannot aspire to become veterinarians— because of a lower grade point average or because circumstances will not allow them to spend the necessary time or money to become veterinarians. Veterinary technicians can also strive to become hospital managers, teachers, or technicians in industry, positions that usually pay well in terms of salary and benefits.

Some things are more important than money. Often an individual profits personally from attending college and successfully completing the requirements for a degree, regardless of what that degree is. These individuals develop more confidence in themselves, which is beneficial for whatever they do in life—parenting, working for a veterinarian, or going on for another degree in a related field.

One of my students, a congenial but somewhat self-effacing mother of three, had never finished high school, had been treated as a person of lesser intelligence most of her life, and had recently been diagnosed as having a learning disorder. It was such an uplift and a joy for me to see this individual, who was actually a person with superior intelligence, gain the confidence not only to complete the program but to really take charge of her life. I like to think that I was a mentor, if not a great teacher, for this young woman and others like her.

Another joy—in the form of a husband—came from Amarillo College. The college had a slogan: "I got my start at Amarillo College." I wanted to amend that jingle to "I got my spouse at Amarillo College." I figured I could recruit as many students, if not more, with my testimony.

George Whiteley was an instructor in the commercial electronics department. We began dating and after six months decided to marry. My last name, "White" became "Whiteley," and I gained another daughter, Sissy, and a son, Rusty.

The day after George and I married, we traveled to Malmstrom Air Force Base located at Great Falls, Montana, for two weeks of military annual training. After the move to Texas, I had become a member of the Army Reserve and served two weeks each year, usually as base veterinarian. George, a retired Air Force master sergeant, seemed to enjoy the reversed role of military spouse. He claimed he was along to serve as my interpreter because he spoke Air Force fluently and I spoke only marginal Army.

When I decided to leave the college and go into practice for myself, George was encouraging and helpful. Working together, we renovated a building behind the house for Cat Clinic. He also helps me by answering the telephone or assisting with patients that need restraint, radiographs, or surgery.

Cat Clinic is designed as a feline house-call service. I travel to clients' homes in a Dodge minivan and transport cats, if necessary, back to the clinic in portable cages.

I enjoy working for myself. Control over what I do and when I do it is important to me. I can arrange my schedule to pick up my daughter after school, and I can make the decision to give myself a day or a week off, if it suits me. By having my hospitalized patients in such proximity, I can monitor their care at all hours of the day or night if necessary. I can also elect to do surgery at midnight if it suits me.

Most everything in life, however, is a trade-off. Working alone takes much time. Except for a woman who answers my telephone in the morning, I do everything myself. Each call is time-consuming. For example, I make three trips in my minivan—to pick up the pet, to deliver it home, and to remove the sutures—for a simple cat spay. I am very accessible to people who want free advice over the telephone or friends who want to stop by and chat. It is easy to get sidetracked by cooking dinner or putting a load of wash in the machine or cleaning the refrigerator.

My veterinary colleagues in Amarillo have been supportive of my practice and often refer patients that need to be seen at home to me, and I reciprocate by referring dogs or cases requiring electrocardiograms or orthopedic surgery to them.

Ten years ago when I practiced in Edmond, Oklahoma, all of my colleagues were men. Today at least ten women veterinarians live near me. Several of us meet for an informal lunch once a week. We discuss cases, read radiographs, and interpret laboratory results. We laugh and moan about the trials and tribulations of animal doctoring. My contact and friendship with these women have given me the confidence to continue in practice.

I designed Cat Clinic to be a limited practice in order to control my time. For more than a decade, I have wanted to write, and I now realize that it requires time and effort to be a good writer. After many years of juggling jobs, children, marriage, and writing, I decided to devote more of that time and effort to the things that are really important to me—family and writing.

I have combined my knowledge of veterinary medicine and my writing goals by starting Professional Veterinary Services, a free-lance public relations business. I write technical literature and articles for private companies and professional magazines. I have public relations and media experience, and I hope to work on a free-lance basis for companies needing a speaker or media spokesperson.

I believe that the purpose of life is to learn and to grow, not to sit back in complacency. Life presents itself sort of like a large schoolroom, and my mission is to try to learn lessons as they are presented.

Sometimes the lessons seem too hard to grasp. For example, one of my practice issues is people who don't pay me. I feel used, rejected, and angry when this happens. Then I may feel guilt for my lack of empathy or compassion. I wish I could say that I have solved this problem, not only for myself but for all the other veterinarians and business people who face the same problem. Yet I realize that the answer will be different for each individual. I am saying no more often to requests from clients who obviously won't pay for one reason or the other. I am working on forgiving and forgetting, but it's slow progress. I think I might have recently graduated from preschool to kindergarten on this particular issue.

I am fortunate that veterinary medicine offers such varied and interesting opportunities. I am easily bored with the same routine and like to wear more than one professional hat. Right now a feline house-call practice and a free-lance writing business in Amarillo, Texas, serve my needs and, hopefully, the needs of clients and patients.

Success is deciding on a goal and making an effort to obtain it. This doesn't mean that goals are carved in stone. Goals change as we change. Who knows what tomorrow will bring? A best-seller, I hope! ■

J

M/